Digestive Diseases

Clinical Reviews

Formerly 'Survey of Digestive Diseases'
Founded in 1983 by T.S.N. Chen and R.K. Zetterman
Former Editor: S.R. Achem (1993–2000)

KARGER

Printed in Switzerland
on acid-free paper by
Reinhardt Druck, Basel

Appears quarterly:
1 volume per year
(4 issues)

Digestive Diseases

General Information

Publication data: 'Digestive Diseases' is published 4 times a year. Volume 25 with 4 issues appears in 2007.

Subscription rates: Subscriptions run for a full calendar year. Prices are given per year.

Personal subscription:

Print or Online	Print/Online combined
CHF 101.00	CHF 146.00
EUR 75.00	EUR 108.00
USD 92.00	USD 133.00
postage and handling	(added to print and print/online)
CHF 23.00 Europe,	CHF 34.20 Overseas
EUR 16.60	
USD 31.40	

Institutional subscription:

Print or Online	Print/Online combined
CHF 1212.00	CHF 1333.00
EUR 898.00	EUR 987.00
USD 1102.00	USD 1212.00
postage and handling	(added to print and print/online)
CHF 28.80 Europe,	CHF 42.80 Overseas
EUR 20.80	
USD 39.20	

Airmail surcharge: CHF 29.00 / USD 26.20
Discount subscription prices:
Please enquire about reduced rates for residents.

Microforms: Please direct all enquiries and orders to:
University Microfilms Inc.
300 North Zeeb Road, P.O. Box 1346
Ann Arbor, MI 48106-1346 (USA)

Subscription orders: Orders can be placed at agencies, bookstores, directly with the Publisher
S. Karger AG, P.O. Box
CH–4009 Basel (Switzerland)
or with any of the following distributors:
Deutschland: S. Karger GmbH, Postfach
D–79095 Freiburg
France: Librairie Luginbühl
36, bd de Latour-Maubourg
F–75007 Paris
Great Britain, Ireland: S. Karger AG
4 Rickett Street
London SW6 1RU, UK
USA: S. Karger Publishers, Inc.
26 West Avon Road, P.O. Box 529
Farmington, CT 06085, USA
India, Bangladesh, Sri Lanka:
Panther Publishers Private Ltd.
33, First Main
Koramangala First Block
Bangalore 560 034, India
Japan: Karger Japan, Inc.
Yushima S Bld. 3F
4-2-3, Yushima, Bunkyo-ku
Tokyo 113-0034, Japan

Change of address: Both old and new address should be sent to the subscription source.

Single issues and back volumes: Information can be obtained through the Publisher.

Advertising: Correspondence and rate requests should be addressed to the Publisher.

Bibliographic indices: This journal is regularly listed in bibliographic services, including *Current Contents®* and Index Medicus/MEDLINE.

Digestive Diseases

Colorectal Cancer

Editors
Christos Dervenis, Athens
Evaghelos Xynos, Heraklion

33 figures and 25 tables, 2007

KARGER
Basel · Freiburg · Paris · London · New York ·
Bangalore · Bangkok · Singapore · Tokyo · Sydney

S. Karger
Medical and Scientific Publishers
Basel • Freiburg • Paris • London
New York • Bangalore • Bangkok
Singapore • Tokyo • Sydney

Disclaimer
The statements, options and data contained in this publication are solely those of the individual authors and contributors and not of the publisher and the editor(s). The appearance of advertisements in the journal is not a warranty, endorsement, or approval of the products or services advertised or of their effectiveness, quality or safety. The publisher and the editor(s) disclaim responsibility for any injury to persons or property resulting from any ideas, methods, instructions or products referred to in the content or advertisements.

Drug Dosage
The authors and the publisher have exerted every effort to ensure that drug selection and dosage set forth in this text are in accord with current recommendations and practice at the time of publication. However, in view of ongoing research, changes in government regulations, and the constant flow of information relating to drug therapy and drug reactions, the reader is urged to check the package insert for each drug for any change in indications and dosage and for added warnings and precautions. This is particularly important when the recommended agent is a new and/or infrequently employed drug.

Printed in Switzerland on acid-free paper by
Reinhardt Druck, Basel
ISBN 978–3–8055–8272–8

KARGER

Fax +41 61 306 12 34
E-Mail karger@karger.ch
www.karger.com

Vol. 25, No. 1, 2007

Digestive Diseases

Contents

KARGER

Fax +41 61 306 12 34
E-Mail karger@karger.ch
www.karger.com

Access to full text and tables of contents, including tentative ones for forthcoming issues: www.karger.com/ddi_issues

Editorial

Digestive Diseases

Dig Dis 2007;25:5–8
DOI: 10.1159/000099165

Rectal Cancer – Towards Establishing a New Strategy of Treatment

Evaghelos Xynos[a] Christos Dervenis[b]

[a]Medical School, University of Crete, Heraklion, and [b]First Department of General Surgery, 'Agia Olga' Hospital, Athens, Greece

During the last three decades, a great deal of progress has been achieved firstly in understanding genetics and natural history, secondly in the establishment of the diagnosis and the accurate staging, and thirdly in the therapeutic modalities of rectal cancer. That progress has led to a substantial improvement in survival and local recurrence rates, greater than that accomplished for colon cancer. Surgery still remains the cornerstone of rectal cancer treatment. The introduction of the concept of total mesorectal excision (TME) by Heald et al. [1], almost 25 years ago, resulted in local recurrence rates of less than 10% [2]. Further to adequate proximal and distal resection bowel margins, TME involves removal of the rectum along with the mesorectal fatty tissue that contains the regional lymph nodes and possible micrometastases covered by an intact rectal fascia propria. In recent years, there has been a debate on the exact anterior plane of dissection while performing a TME. Heald et al. [3] propose that the anterior plane of dissection should run in front of the Denonvilliers' fascia down to the point it fuses with the prostatic capsule, and not between the fascia and the anterior rectal wall. By this approach, which sounds reasonable in an anatomical and oncological sense, the anterior mesorectum of the middle third of the rectum covered by the Denonvilliers' fascia is removed. It is of great importance that both the surgeon and the pathologist evaluate macroscopically and classify the completeness of the rectal cancer resection specimen. Quality control of surgery provides the first prognostic information concerning local and distant recurrence [4, 5].

With such impressive results of local control and survival after TME, adjuvant radiotherapy and chemotherapy seem to offer no additional benefit. However, there are always patients at risk to develop local recurrence and distant metastases. These subsets include patients with lymph node metastases, venous or lymphatic vessels invasion, distally located tumors most likely requiring an abdominoperineal resection (APR) and, most importantly, a threatened by tumor extension circumferential margin of resection (CRM). It is established beyond any doubt that the status of the CRM is possibly the strongest predictive factor of local recurrence or even survival. A positive CRM, namely presence of tumor at a distance <1 mm from the CRM on the fixed specimen, is associated with local recurrence rates significantly greater than those seen in patients with negative CRM [4, 6, 7]. To improve surgical treatment outcomes in patients with extensive rectal tumors, neoadjuvant radiotherapy has been applied in order to downstage the disease. According to the Dutch Colorectal Cancer Group randomized trial [8], hypofractionated 5 Gy/day for 5 days radiother-

KARGER

Fax +41 61 306 12 34
E-Mail karger@karger.ch
www.karger.com

0257–2753/07/0251–0005$23.50/0

Accessible online at:
www.karger.com/ddi

Assoc. Prof. E. Xynos
Medical School, University of Crete
19, Michelidaki Str.
GR–71202 Heraklion, Crete (Greece)
Tel. +30 2810 280 002, Fax +30 2810 280 009, E-Mail exynos@gmail.com

apy followed by TME 7–10 days later offers local recurrence rates well below 5% as compared to TME alone. The main message of the trial is that a multimodality therapeutic approach depending on the stage of the disease would optimize the results of TME. Several studies [9–12] propose the preoperative application of a full radiation scheme of 45–60 Gy over a period of 5 weeks, concomitantly accompanied by chemotherapy, and followed by TME approximately 10 weeks later. According to the results of those studies, neoadjuvant chemoradiation not only downstages but also downsizes the disease, rendering feasible an R0 resection of an otherwise locally extended and possibly not resectable rectal tumor, offering better local recurrence and survival rates and possibly preserving the anal sphincters. However, there are still numerous questions seeking answers, questions concerning the optimal tailoring of the neoadjuvant treatment according to stage and histological characteristics of the tumor, the optimal imaging modality of final staging prior to surgery, the time interval between end of chemoradiation and surgery, the histopathological assessment of the primary tumor, lymph nodes and CRM on the fixed surgical specimen, and the functional outcome. Furthermore, under the light of neoadjuvant treatment, the place of adjuvant chemotherapy and additional radiotherapy should be redefined. The CR07 multicentric randomized trial, which has been recently completed, attempts to answer some of the aforementioned questions. According to the results of the trial, administration of neoadjuvant short course radiotherapy followed by TME is associated with significantly lower local recurrence and higher survival rates compared to TME alone that is followed by adjuvant chemoradiotherapy only in T3, T4 and node-positive cases. This stands true for all rectal tumors including T1 and T2 as well as tumors located in the proximal-endoperitoneal third of the rectum [pers. commun.].

It is conceivable that preoperative staging is of paramount importance for the staging of the disease and, in particular, for assessing extension of the primary tumor and status of regional lymph nodes. Imaging modalities, including magnetic resonance imaging, spiral computed tomography and endoanal ultrasonography, complement each other to offer pretreatment accurate staging rates well over 90% [13]. Furthermore, it is imperative that specific imaging definitions must be further elaborated so as to improve staging of the rectal cancer after neoadjuvant chemoradiotherapy.

There is nowadays a trend towards performing more sphincter-preserving operations than APR for tumors located in the lower third of the rectum. All trials reported that radiotherapy should be given prior to surgery, in order to reduce the stage and the size of the tumor [14–16]. Some authors [17] even recommend neoadjuvant long-course chemoradiotherapy even for stage I tumors, although there are reports according to which, despite downsizing, neoadjuvant long-course chemoradiotherapy does not seem to increase the sphincter-preserving operation rate compared to preoperative short-course radiation for T3–T4 low rectal tumors [18]. However, the concept that tumor downsizing and increase in the macroscopic distance between the lower edge of the tumor and the anorectal ring facilitates low resections and anastomoses may be hazardous; there might be microscopic tumor deposits distal to the macroscopic lower edge of the tumor and a compromise in distal clearance of the rectal wall, thus increasing the risk of anastomotic recurrence. Therefore, it is recommended that the decision to perform a sphincter-sparing operation should be taken prior to the neoadjuvant treatment. Depending on the type of resection, conventional low anterior or intersphincteric, the colo-anal anastomosis is fashioned either with the use of stapling devices or by hand-sawing. Intersphincteric resection may be applied to tumors located almost even in the anal canal, provided the sphincters are not invaded. In this case the colon in a form of a pouch is anastomosed by hand to the anoderm [19].

Although more sphincter-preserving operations are attempted, APR is still applied, apparently following new specific indications. An increased risk of local and distant recurrence after an APR compared to low anterior resection of the rectum has been reported. This is attributed to the low level and the unfavorable characteristics of the tumor, as well as the increased incidence of positive CRM, rather than the type of the operation itself. Related to the depth of invasion, very low rectal tumors tend to spread laterally and downwards to the lateral pelvic wall lymph nodes. Hence, in this case the criterion of a free CRM is not satisfied by TME only. In other words, a resection specimen involving the whole mesorectum and the anal sphincters creating a sort of 'waist' in between them is not of adequate quality. On the high-quality specimen after an APR, there should appear a part of the rectosacral fascia with the mesorectum above and the plate of the lavatory muscles below, in the form of a 'cylinder' [20, 21]. At present however, there are no strong data supporting the view that a 'cylindrical' APR specimen is associated with less recurrence and better survival rates than the conventional one in the form of a 'waist'. In any case, it is suggested that low rectal tumors should be treated rather aggressively by adding preoperative chemoradiation more often than in higher rectal tumors.

Recently, surgery for rectal cancer can also be accomplished by laparoscopy. At present, the results published show that the approach is safe in terms of postoperative morbidity and mortality. The quality of the specimen is comparable to that after conventional surgery. Because of the better view into the pelvis, there is a feeling among the surgeons practicing laparoscopy that a R0 resection for rectal cancer is easier, safer and more complete by laparoscopy than by the open approach. However, strong evidence concerning local recurrence and survival is still awaited [22]. Several technical problems, such us proper distal transection of the rectum in obese male patients, also have to be resolved by improvement of instrumentation.

For rectal tumors with minimal invasion of the bowel wall, local excision by means of the transanal endoscopic microsurgery (TEM) device has been attempted. T1 tumors are usually excised by this approach, although there is a report of TEM for T2 rectal tumors after a short course of preoperative radiotherapy with a local recurrence rate of 5%. However, data derived from some series show that TEM, even for T1 tumor, fails to match the good results acquired after abdominal surgery, in terms of recurrence [23]. Possibly, a multimodality approach, including neoadjuvant treatment, may improve the long-term results of TEM.

Several ongoing trials aim towards offering plausible answers to most of the above questions and setting new guidelines for a multimodality treatment of rectal cancer with even further improved recurrence and survival rates and quality of life. Furthermore, multidisciplinary approach requires not only close collaboration between the surgeon, the pathologist, the radiologist and the oncologist, but also core training of the team.

In the present issue of *Digestive Disease*, most of the current knowledge and trends in the treatment of rectal cancer is gathered and presented in reviews. Also, in a review of the molecular biological changes characterizing colorectal cancer, the possible implementations of genetic studies in screening and follow-up is discussed. Finally, the issue includes original articles which focus on several aspects of the management of patients with colorectal cancer.

References

1 Heald RJ, Husband EM, Ryall RDH: The mesorectum in rectal cancer surgery – the clue to pelvic recurrence? Br J Surg 1982;69:613–616.

2 MacFarlane JK, Ryall RDH, Heald RJ: Mesorectal excision for rectal cancer. Lancet 1993; 341:457–460.

3 Heald RJ, Moran BJ, Brown G, Daniels IR: Optimal total mesorectal excision for rectal cancer is by dissection in front of Denonvillier's fascia. Br J Surg 2004;91:121–123.

4 Nagtegaal ID, van de Velde CJH, van der Worp E, Kapiteijn E, Quirke P, van Krieken JHJM, Dutch Colorectal Cancer Group: Macroscopic evaluation of the rectal cancer resection specimen: clinical significance of the pathologist in quality control. J Clin Oncol 2002;20:1729–1734.

5 Quirke P: Training and quality assurance for rectal cancer: 20 years of data is enough. Lancet (Oncol) 2003;4:695–702.

6 Nagtegaal ID, Marijnen CA, Kranenbarg EK: Circumferential margins involvement is still an important predictor of local recurrence in rectal carcinoma: not one millimeter but two millimeters is the limit. Am J Surg Pathol 2002;26:350–357.

7 Wibe A, Rendedal PR, Svensson E: Prognostic significance of the circumferential resection margin following total mesorectal excision for rectal cancer. Br J Surg 2002;89: 327–334.

8 Kapiteijn E, Marijnen CA, Nagtegaal ID: Preoperative radiotherapy combined with total mesorectal excision for resectable rectal cancer. N Engl J Med 2001;345:638–646.

9 Rodel C, Marus P, Papadopoulos T, et al: Prognostic significance of tumour regression after preoperative chemoradiotherapy for rectal cancer. J Clin Oncol 2005;23:8688–8696.

10 Chan AK, Wong A, Jenken D, et al: Posttreatment TNM staging is a prognostic indicator of survival and recurrence in tethered or fixed rectal carcinoma after preoperative chemotherapy and radiotherapy. Int J Radiat Oncol Biol Phys 2005;1: 665–677.

11 Pucciarelli S, Toppan P, Friso ML, et al: Complete pathologic response following preoperative chemoradiation therapy for middle to lower rectal cancer is not a prognostic factor for better outcome. Dis Colon Rectum 2004;47:798–807.

12 Bossett JF, Calsis G, Mineur L, et al: Enhanced tumouricidal effect of chemotherapy with preoperative radiotherapy for rectal cancer. Preliminary results EORTC 22921. J Clin Oncol 2005;24:5620–5627.

13 Brown G, Radcliffe AG, Newcombe RG, et al: Preoperative assessment of prognostic factors in rectal cancer using high-resolution magnetic resonance imaging. Br J Surg 2003; 90:355–364.

14 Crane CH, Skibber JM, Feig BW, et al: Response to preoperative chemoradiation increases the use of sphincter-preserving surgery in patients with locally advanced low rectal carcinoma. Cancer 2003;97:517–524.

15 Kuvshinoff B, Maghfoor I, Miedema B, et al: Distal margin requirements after operative chemoradiotherapy for distal rectal carcinomas: are < or = 1 cm distal margin sufficient? Ann Surg Oncol 2000;8:163–169.

16 Rouanet P, Saint-Aubert B, Lemansky B, et al: Restorative and nonrestorative surgery for low rectal carcinoma after high-dose radiation. Dis Colon Rectum 2002;45:305–315.

17 Mohiuddin M, Regine WF, Marks GJ, Marks JW: High-dose preoperative radiation and the challenge of sphincter-preservation surgery for cancer of the distal 2 cm of the rectum. Int J Radiat Oncol Biol Phys 1998;40:569–574.
18 Bujko K, Nowacki MP, Nasierowska-Guttmejer A, et al: Sphincter preservation following preoperative radiotherapy for rectal cancer: report of a randomized trial comparing short-term radiotherapy vs. conventionally fractionated radiochemotherapy. Radiother Oncol 2004;72:15–24.
19 Rullier E, Goffe B, Bonnel C, Zerbib F, Caudri M, Saric J: Preoperative radiochemotherapy and sphincter-saving resection for T3 carcinomas of the lower third of the rectum. Ann Surg 2001;234:633–640.
20 Wibe A, Syse A, Andersen E, Tretli S, Myrvold HE, Soreide O on behalf of the Norwegian Rectal Cancer Group: Oncological outcomes after total mesorectal excision for cure for cancer of the lower rectum: anterior vs. abdominoperineal resection. Dis Colon Rectum 2004;47:48–58.
21 Radcliffe A: Can the results of anorectal (abdominoperineal resection) be improved: are circumferential resection margins too often positive? Colorectal Dis 2006;8:160–167.
22 Guillou PJ, Quirke P, Thorpe H, et al.: Short-term endpoints of conventional versus laparoscopic assisted surgery in patients with colorectal cancer (MRC CLASICC trial): multicentre, randomised controlled trial. Lancet 2005;365:1718–1726.
23 Lezoche E, Guerrieri M, Paganini AM, et al: Transanal endoscopic versus total mesorectal laparoscopic resections of T2-N0 low rectal cancers after neoadjuvant treatment: a prospective randomized trial with a 3-year minimum follow-up period. Surg Endosc 2005;19:751–756.

Review Article

Digestive Diseases

Dig Dis 2007;25:9–19
DOI: 10.1159/000099166

Genetic Alterations in Sporadic and Hereditary Colorectal Cancer: Implementations for Screening and Follow-Up

John Souglakos

Department of Medical Oncology, University General Hospital of Heraklion, Heraklion, Greece

Key Words
Attenuated familial adenomatous polyposis · Familial adenomatous polyposis · Familial juvenile polyposis · Hereditary colorectal cancer · Hereditary non-polyposis colorectal cancer · Juvenile polyposis coli · MYH polyposis syndrome · Peutz-Jeghers syndrome · Sporadic colorectal cancer

Abstract
The genetics underlying an inherited predisposition to cancer are rapidly being uncovered. This fact may ultimately lead to the routine use of molecular tools to diagnose these disorders, and establish interventions to prevent the development of cancer. Among the multiple cancer family syndromes, several are known to be associated with the development of colon cancer. These disorders may be diagnosed during evaluation of the index patient or during screening of family members who are at risk. Although the effectiveness of screening and surveillance strategies is unproven in controlled clinical trials for any of these syndromes, the high cancer risk warrants screening, and reasonable recommendations can be made. Several other genetic syndromes are associated with gastrointestinal polyposis. The risk of colon cancer in these diseases is uncertain, and may not be increased and they are not mentioned in this review. Examples include Cowden disease, intestinal ganglioneuromatosis, Ruvalcaba-Myhre-Smith syndrome, Devon family syndrome, and Cronkite-Canada syndrome.

Introduction

Colorectal cancer (CRC) is a major cause of morbidity and mortality worldwide. CRC is the third most common cancer and the third leading cause of cancer death in both sexes, accounting for approximately 10% of cancer deaths overall [1]. The lifetime incidence for patients at average risk is 5%, with 90% of cases occurring after age 50. Approximately 1 in 3 people who develop CRC die of this disease. While early stage CRC is frequently curable with surgery, unresectable metastatic disease is a fatal disease. These facts indicate the crucial role of an effective screening and follow-up programs in order to identify the disease in early stages. Furthermore, the identification of premalignant lesions is a prerequisite to effective CRC.

The risk factors for CRC are both environmental and genetic. These different risk factors reflect the mode of presentation of CRC that follows one of the following three: sporadic, inherited, and familial. Sporadic disease, in which there is no family history, accounts for approximately 70% of all CRC. The patients are usually older than 50 years of age and dietary and environmental factors have been etiologically implicated, although genetic changes which lead to the adenoma-carcinoma sequence have been described [2]. Less than 10% of patients have an inherited predisposition to CRC, and these cases are subdivided according to whether or not colonic polyps are a major disease manifestation. The diseases with polyposis include familial adenomatous polyposis (FAP) [3], and the hamartomatous polyposis syndromes (e.g.,

KARGER
Fax +41 61 306 12 34
E-Mail karger@karger.ch
www.karger.com

0257–2753/07/0251–0009$23.50/0

Accessible online at:
www.karger.com/ddi

Dr. John Souglakos, MD, PhD
Department of Medical Oncology
University General Hospital of Heraklion, PO Box 1352
GR–71110 Heraklion (Greece)
Tel./Fax +30 2810 392 802, E-Mail johnsougl@gmail.com

Table 1. CRC predisposition genes

Gene (synonyms)[a]	Syndrome	Hereditary pattern	Second hit	Pathway[b]	Tumor types[c]
Tumor suppressor genes					
APC	FAP	Dominant	Inactivation of WT allele	APC	Colon, thyroid, stomach, intestine
AXIN2	Attenuated FAP	Dominant	Inactivation of WT allele	APC	Colon
BMPR1A	Juvenile polyposis	Dominant	Inactivation of WT allele	SMAD	Gastrointestinal
SMAD4 (*DPC4*)	Juvenile polyposis	Dominant	Inactivation of WT allele	SMAD	Gastrointestinal
Stability genes					
MUTYH	Attenuated polyposis	Recessive	?	BER	Colon
MSH2,MLH1, MSH6, PMS2	HNPCC	Dominant	Inactivation of WT allele	MMR	Colon, uterus
Oncogenes					

WT = Wild type.
[a] Representative genes of all the major pathways and hereditary cancer predisposition types are listed. Approved gene symbols are provided for each entry, with alternative names in parentheses.
[b] In many cases, the gene has been implicated in several pathways.
[c] In most cases, the non-familial tumor spectrum caused by somatic mutations of the gene includes those occurring in the familial cases plus additional tumor types.

Peutz-Jeghers, juvenile polyposis) [4], while those without polyposis include hereditary non-polyposis colorectal cancer (HNPCC, Lynch syndrome I), and the cancer family syndrome (Lynch syndrome II) [5]. These conditions are associated with a high risk of developing CRC, and the genetic mutations underlying many of them have been identified. The third and least well understood pattern is known as 'familial' CRC. Up to 25% of affected patients have a family history of CRC, but the pattern is not consistent with one of the inherited syndromes described above. Individuals from these families are at increased risk of developing CRC, although the risk is not as high as with the inherited syndromes. It was proposed that this group of patients represents individuals with genetic changes with an autosomal recessive pattern of inheritance. Indeed the discovery that biallelic mutations of the base excision repair gene, *MYH*, resulted in an increased risk of colorectal adenomas and cancer led to the first description of an autosomal recessive cancer syndrome [6].

The revolution in cancer research has proven that cancer is a genetic disease. The elucidation of human genome sequence has made it possible to identify genetic alterations in cancer in unprecedented detail [7]. The initial genetic alterations of a cell that triggers its aberrant proliferation are followed by the accumulation of additional mutations among its progeny. Finally, a selection process occurred by which subclones with enhanced growth properties become dominant within the tumor, a process that was called tumor progression [8]. A clear histologic and molecular genetics evolution from precancerous lesions to flunky malignant and invasive cancer has been defined for the majority of cases of CRC [9–11].

Major Genetic Alterations CRC

Alterations in three types of genes are responsible for tumorigenesis in CRC as well as in the other tumor types: oncogenes, tumor suppressor genes and stability genes (tables 1, 2) [12]. The carcinogenesis in colon epithelium is a multistep process. In 1990, Fearon and Vogelstein [9] described the molecular basis for CRC as a multistep process in which each accumulated genetic event conferred a selective growth advantage to the colonic epithelial cell. According to the Vogelstein model, also known as the adenoma-carcinoma sequence, germline or somatic mutations are required for malignant transformation, and it is the accumulation of multiple genetic mutations rather than their sequence that determines the biological behavior of the tumor (fig. 1). Germline mutations underlie the common inherited syndromes (e.g., APC, HNPCC), while sporadic cancers

Table 2. Genes that are mutated somatically but not inherited in mutant form

Gene (synonyms)[a]	Somatic mutation type[b]	Cancers with mutant gene[c]	Pathway
CTNNB1 (β-catenin)	Activating codon change	Colon, liver, medulloblastomas	APC
BAX	Inactivating codon change	Colon, stomach	APOP
FBXW7 (*CDC4*)	Inactivating codon change	Colon, uterine, ovarian, breast	CIN
PI3KCA	Activating codon change	Colon, stomach, brain, breast	PI3K
BRAF	Activating codon change	Melanoma, colorectal, thyroid	RTK
FES	Activating codon change	Colon	RTK
KRAS2, N-RAS	Activating codon change	Colorectal, pancreatic, non-small cell lung cancer	RTK
NTRK1, 3	Translocation, activating codon change	Thyroid, secretory breast, colon	RTK
SMAD2	Inactivating codon change	Colon, breast	SMAD
TGFBR1, TGFBR2	Inactivating codon change	Colon, stomach, ovarian	SMAD
HOXD11, 13; HOX11, HOX11L2			
MAP2K4 (*MKK4*)	Inactivating codon change	Pancreas, breast, colon	Unknown
PTNP1, 11	Activating codon change	Leukemias, colon	Unknown

[a] Representative genes of all the major pathways and cancer types are listed. Approved gene symbols are provided for each entry, with alternative names in parentheses.
[b] Activating codon change, intragenic mutation altering one or a small number of base pairs that activates the gene product, indicating that it is an oncogene; inactivating codon change, any mutation (point mutation, small or large deletion, etc.) that inactivates the gene product, indicating that the gene is a tumor suppressor. Amplifications and translocations generally affect oncogenes, though occasional translocations disrupt a gene rather than activate it.
[c] Only representative types of cancers are listed when a gene is mutated in many tumor types.

result from the stepwise accumulation of multiple somatic mutations.

Indeed, it was well known for many years that most CRCs arise from pre-existing adenomas, usually as result of mutation in the adenomatous polyposis coli *(APC)* gene [13] and are characterized by chromosomal instability [10]. However, approximately 10–15% of CRC arise via the microsatellite instability (MSI, mutator, DNA replication error) [11, 14, 15]. These two types of colorectal carcinogenesis present a range of distinctive genetic, pathologic and clinical characteristics [16–18].

Tumors with chromosomal instability are associated with hyperploidity, allelic losses (17p, 18q, 8p, 22q), frequent tumor suppressor gene mutations (p53 and APC), are mainly located in the left colon and were correlated with an unfavorable outcome.

Mutations in the *APC* gene, which are a feature common to both inherited and sporadic tumors, occur early in the process, followed by mutation in the *k-ras* gene while mutations of the p53 suppressor gene generally occur late in the process [19]. *APC* represent the most critical gene in the early development of CRC is the *APC* tumor suppressor gene. Germline mutations of the *APC* gene are responsible for the F somatic mutations in both alleles are present in almost 80% of sporadic CRC. The function of the APC protein and the mechanism whereby the abnormal gene promotes tumor formation are beginning to be understood [20, 21]. Loss of function mutations in the *APC* or activating mutations in the β-*catenin* gene result in the nuclear accumulation of β-catenin, which binds and activates the transcription factor T-cell factor (Tcf)-4 [22]. It is proposed that β-catenin/Tcf-4 acts as a switch controlling proliferation versus differentiation in the intestinal crypt epithelial cells [23].

An important clue was the observation that most sporadic CRC with normal or wild-type *APC* had mutations in β-catenin, a protein involved in the same signaling cascade as *APC*, the Wnt (wingless-type) signaling pathway [23, 24]. The recognition of the importance of the *APC* gene began with genetic studies linking inheritance of the FAP syndrome to chromosome 5q21, and the subsequent identification of germline mutations involving a gene at this locus, the *APC* gene. The earliest malignant lesions in these patients, dysplastic aberrant crypt foci (microadenomas) and small adenomatous polyps, have lost the second APC allele (through deletion or somatic mutation), suggesting that APC loss is a very early event in colorectal tumorigenesis.

A germline mutation in codon 1307 in the *APC* gene, also named as I1307K *APC* mutation, has been described

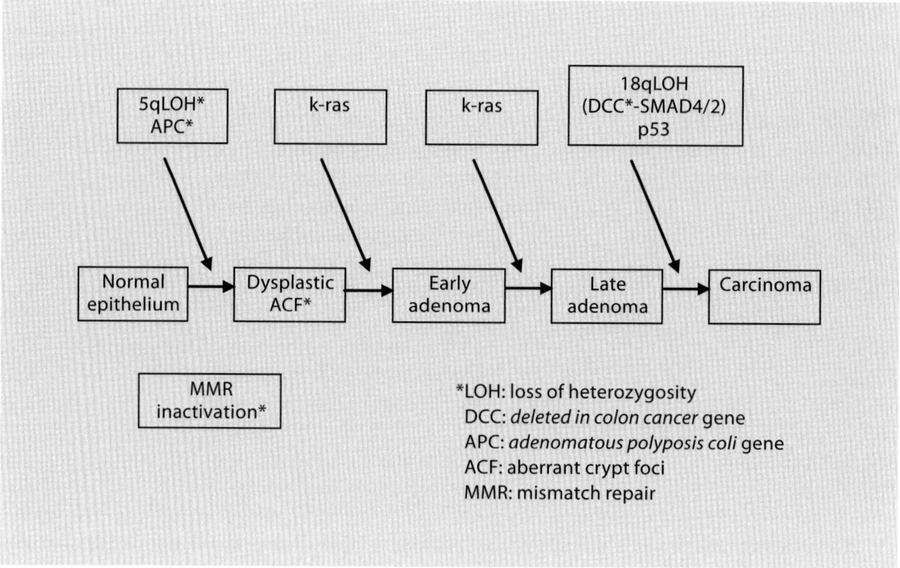

Fig. 1. Adenoma-carcinoma sequence.

in Ashkenazi Jewish individuals and has been linked with familial CRC [25, 26]. The mutation is found in 6% of all persons of Ashkenazi Jewish descent, but in a higher frequency of Ashkenazi Jews with both a personal and family history of CRC (28%) [25]. This mutation was previously thought to represent a polymorphism because it does not cause protein structure abnormalities, but creates a small hypermutable region of the gene, which predisposes to the development of carcinomas [25]. The relative risk for CRC, although elevated relative to the general population, is much lower in affected individuals compared to those with FAP.

The *ras* oncogene exists as three cellular variants: *H-ras, K-ras,* and *N-ras.* Although all three oncogenes, when mutated, have the ability to transform normal cells, *K-ras* is the most frequently mutated in human CRC [27]. The ras oncogenes encode a family of small proteins with homology to G-proteins that regulate cellular signal transduction by acting as a one-way switch for the transmission of extracellular growth signals to the nucleus [28]. *Ras* mutations are found in up to 50% of sporadic CRCs, and 50% of colonic adenomas >1 cm; they are rarely seen in smaller adenomas [2]. The lack of mutations in smaller adenomas suggests that ras mutations are acquired during later adenoma progression [29].

The *p53* gene on chromosome 17p is the most commonly mutated gene in human cancer. Loss of heterozygosity (LOH) in the 17p locus could be identified in up to 75% of CRCs, while they are rarely lost in adenomas and aberrant crypt foci, suggesting that p53 loss represents a relatively late event in colorectal tumorigenesis [2, 9, 30].

As with p53 and the APC gene, the first evidence of a tumor suppressor gene on chromosome 18q came from studies of allelic loss in CRC. In an early study, one copy of 18q was lost in 73% of sporadic CRC and 47% of large adenomas with foci of invasive cancer, but in fewer than 15% of less advanced adenomas [2].

In 1989, a candidate gene termed the *'deleted in colon cancer' (DCC)* gene was identified at 18q21, and point mutations in the *DCC* gene have been identified in CRC [31, 32]. A second tumor suppressor gene at 18q was identified termed *SMAD. SMAD4* encodes a protein that may be important to the signaling pathway of the transforming growth factor-β (TGF-β) superfamily of signaling polypeptides. TGF-β suppresses the growth of most normal cells, and many cancer cells are resistant to this growth-suppressive effect [33]. Mutations in *SMAD4* or a third putative tumor suppressor gene that also maps to 18q *(SMAD2)* have been found in a subset of sporadic CRC [34]. Germline mutations in the SMAD4 gene have been identified as the causative mutation in some affected families with familial juvenile polyposis (FJP) [35]. The PTEN gene coding for a phosphatase and the BMPR1A gene coding for a serine-threonine kinase receptor have also been linked to FJP in some families [36]. The mechanism by which these mutations cause hamartomas is not understood, but genetic testing is now becoming available for these syndromes.

Peutz-Jeghers syndrome, another hamartomas polyposis syndrome, has been linked to germline mutations of *LKB1* (located on chromosome 19p), which encodes the serine-threonine kinase STK-11 [37]. Among their multiple functions, STK-11 can regulate p53-mediated apoptosis [38]. In addition, adenosine monophosphate-activated protein kinase has been identified as being a direct phosphorylation target for LKB1, implicating LKB1 in the control of cellular metabolism [39, 40].

On the other hand, tumors with MSI are euploid tumors without allelic losses, present infrequent tumor suppressor gene mutations *(p53 and APC)* and more frequently mutations of the *TGBβ-RII, BAX, TCF4, Caspase 5, HIF1α,* and oncogene mutation *(BRAF* and *PI3KCA)*, and are located mainly in the proximal colon, have a greater mucinous component, contain lymphocytic infiltration, and are more often poorly differentiated. Despite the latter feature, the presence of MSI is associated with longer survival in both HNPCC and sporadic cases [41].

Mismatch repair (MMR) genes are responsible for correcting the ubiquitous nucleotide base mispairs and small insertions or deletions that occur during DNA replication [42]. Several of these genes have been identified, including *hMSH2 (human mutS homolog 2), hMLH1 (human mutL homolog 1), hPMS1* and *hPMS2 (human post-meiotic segregation 1 and 2), hMSH6 (human mutS homolog 6),* and *hMLH3*, a mismatch repair gene that interacts with *MLH1.*

HNPCC is caused due to germline mutations in one of the MMR genes. MMR gene deficiencies can also be found in approximately 10–15% of sporadic CRCs [41]. However, sporadic tumors with defective MMR do not contain MMR gene mutations, instead they have epigenetic changes that silence gene expression [43].

Cells with MMR deficiency accumulate DNA errors throughout the genome [11]. The biologic 'footprint' of an MMR defect is the accumulation of abnormalities in short sequences of nucleotide bases that are repeated dozens to hundreds of times within the genome – these are called microsatellites [11]. Several critical growth regulatory genes (e.g., the transforming growth factor-β type II receptor, BAX, the insulin-like growth factor II receptor) contain microsatellites in the promoter region and are therefore susceptible to frameshift mutations. This leaves the cell vulnerable to mutations in these genes controlling cell growth. As abnormalities in the microsatellites are common with MMR deficiency, this phenomenon is termed microsatellite instability (MSI) [44].

Germline mutations in the base excision repair gene *mutY homolog (MYH)* have been described in a small proportion of patients with multiple colorectal adenomas and a family history of CRC [45, 46]. Sometimes *(MYH)* mutations coexist in conjunction with somatic mutations in the APC gene [47]. These mutations predispose patients to recessive inheritance of multiple colonic adenomas, and the phenotype of classic adenomatous polyposis. In one series of 152 patients with multiple adenomas seen at one institution, 7.5% of those without a germline APC mutation were found to have two separate germline MYH mutations [45]. More importantly, an increasing number of reports suggest that germline mutations in these MYH genes may account for a substantial fraction of familial CRCs that occur in the absence of a dominantly inherited familial syndrome [48–50].

The genetic changes underlying an inherited predisposition to cancer are rapidly being uncovered, which may ultimately permit the routine use of molecular tools to diagnose these disorders, and the use of screening strategies and interventions to prevent the development of cancer.

Guidelines for Screening and Follow-Up

Before deciding how to screen, clinicians should decide whether the individual patient is at average or increased risk. A few simple questions are all that is necessary: Do you have a family history of CRC? If so, in first-degree relatives, at what age of onset, and how many? Have you had a personal history of CRC or adenomatous polyps?

The patient is considered average risk if the answer to all these questions is 'no'. Patients answering yes to any of these questions need to be evaluated further. These questions should be asked well before the patient would ordinarily begin screening (at age 50 years) if he or she were at average risk because screening should begin earlier for patients with increased risk conditions.

Familial Adenomatous Polyposis and Attenuated Familial Adenomatous Polyposis

Classic FAP is characterized by the development of multiple colonic adenomas during the early teenage years with progressive increase so that hundreds to thousands of polyps are recognized by adulthood. Colonic adenomas are observed approximately 10–15 years after the appearance of polyposis, and almost always by the age of 40 years. FAP-associated adenomas and adenocarcinomas are distributed through the entire colon and are histologically identical to those found in the sporadic CRC. Gastric polyps can develop and are typically benign funding gland adenomas, although gastric adenocarcinomas have also been observed in FAP families from Korea and Japan [1]. Duodenal, periampullary, or ampullary adenomas eventually develop in nearly all FAP patients. Approximately 10% will develop duodenal adenocarcinoma by the age of 60, making it the second most common malignancy in FAP [2].

Extraintestinal features include desmoid tumors, epidermoid cysts, osteosarcomas, follicular and papillary thyroid tumors, congenital hypertrophy of the retinal pigmented epithelium, and rarely hepatoblastomas and retinoblastomas. Turcot's syndrome refers to familial CRC with central nervous system tumors. Medulloblastomas have been associated with FAP, whereas glioblastomas are primarily seen in HNPCC kindreds.

An attenuated version of FAP (AFAP) differs from the classic form in that there are substantially fewer colonic polyps (<100). These polyps tend to develop on the right side of the colon and the average ages at which colorectal polyps and cancer occur are delayed approximately 15 years. The features of AFAP can also overlap with HNPCC [3], and genetic testing can distinguish between two syndromes.

Germline mutations of the *APC* gene are located throughout the entire gene, and more than 90% of mutations introduce a premature stop codon that results in a truncated protein product [4]. Certain genotype-phenotype correlations have been identified. Classic FAP is seen with mutations located in the central region between codons 169 and 1393 and mutations between codons 1250 and 1464 have been associated with particularly severe polyposis [5].

Family members of patients with classic FAP, Gardner's syndrome, or Turcot's syndrome should be offered genetic counseling and testing if appropriate. At-risk children should usually be offered genetic testing around age 10–12. Genetic testing is not recommended in children prior to age 10 because it would not lead to a change in clinical care and may lead to problems with parental bonding, peer rejection, and poor self-image.

Gene carriers or at-risk family members who have not had genetic testing or are from families in whom the gene test is uninformative should be offered a flexible sigmoidoscopy or colonoscopy every 12 months starting at around age 10–12 and continuing until age 35–40 if negative. Classic FAP almost always involves the rectosigmoid so that sigmoidoscopy alone is adequate but many pediatric gastroenterologists screen with colonoscopy.

Screening of the upper gastrointestinal tract with upper endoscopy for gastric and duodenal polyps has been recommended [6], although the benefit has not been proven in clinical trials. A baseline examination with both an end- and side-viewing endoscope is recommended upon diagnosis, and repeated every 3–5 years. The development of symptoms referable to the upper digestive tract, including pancreatitis or signs or symptoms related to biliary obstruction, should prompt a repeat investigation at an earlier interval.

The British Society of Gastroenterology recommends upper gastrointestinal surveillance every 3 years from age 30 and more frequently if there is extensive polyposis [7]. Other authorities recommend frequent surveillance and targeted endoscopic treatment (adjusted by severity of duodenal lesions), but acknowledge that these modalities alone cannot guarantee a polyp-free duodenum [8].

Adenomas identified in the duodenum or the papilla of Vater should be removed endoscopically if possible, and follow-up examination should be performed yearly [9]. An abnormal appearing papilla should be biopsied, since adenomas in the duodenum have a predilection for the papilla. Some authorities also recommend obtaining routine biopsies of the papilla, even if it appears grossly normal.

Once colonic polyposis is established in a gene carrier or an at-risk member of an FAP family, a full colonoscopy should be performed to evaluate the extent of the colonic polyposis. An initial upper endoscopic examination should also be performed and a consultation should be arranged to discuss the timing of a colectomy. The number, size, and worst histology of the colonic adenomas determine the optimal timing of colectomy.

Colectomy at the time of initial diagnosis is strongly recommended in patients with multiple large (>1 cm) adenomas or adenomas with villous histology and/or high-grade dysplasia and is the safest approach of all those with profuse polyposis at initial diagnosis. Patients in the second decade of life with only sparse, small (<5 mm) adenomas can usually be followed endoscopically with surgery scheduled to accommodate school and work schedules. Some centers try to allow such patients to finish high school if the endoscopic appearance of the colon is stable, to minimize the psychological trauma of a colectomy during adolescence. The preferred operation in children is a total proctocolectomy with ileoanal anastomosis. A subtotal colectomy with ongoing surveillance or a total colectomy is reasonable in patients with attenuated adenomatous polyposis who have little rectal involvement. If rectum is left intact, rigorous follow-up with sigmoidectomy every 6–12 months is required.

The risk of colon adenocarcinoma in classic FAP approaches 100% by age 45. Colonoscopy is not effective for identifying polyps with advanced pathology or in detecting early cancers, because the presence of multiple polyps precludes adequate sampling. Although the non-steroidal anti-inflammatory drug sulindac can cause regression of colorectal adenomas in FAP, regression of polyps is incomplete, and the degree of protection from the development of CRC is unknown. Sulindac (75 or 150 mg twice daily) was ineffective in delaying the time of initial development of adenomas in a controlled trial involving 41 proven FAP gene carriers [12]. Thus, sulindac is unlikely to replace colectomy as primary therapy for FAP but it is being used in some centers to slow the development of adenomas prior to colectomy and to delay new polyp formation in the rectum after subtotal colectomy [13]. One of the COX-2 inhibitors (celecoxib) was approved by the FDA based upon a controlled trial involving 77 patients in which it was associated with a 28% reduction in the number of polyps [14].

Hereditary Non-Polyposis Colorectal Cancer

Among the colon cancer syndromes, HNPCC is the most common and accounts for close to 1% of the CRC in the USA [10] and nearly 2% in Europe [11]. The lifetime risk for the development of CRC in affected individuals is 80%. The average age at diagnosis of CRC is 45 years. A unique set of extracolonic tumors in associated with HNPCC (table 3).

Clinical criteria for the diagnosis of HNPCC take into account the age of diagnosis of CRC, the number of affected family members, and the presence of extracolonic tumors. The Amsterdam I criteria of 1990 [51] are considered to be highly specific for the diagnosis of HNPCC. The modified Amsterdam and Amsterdam II criteria [52] were proposed in order to provide less stringent guidelines. In 1996, the Bethesda guidelines [53] were formulated to encompass an even broader spectrum of at risk patients, thereby maximizing sensitivity but necessarily reducing specificity. These criteria were updated and simplified in 2004 [54].

A consortium of experts has developed guidelines for cancer surveillance in patients diagnosed with HNPCC. These recommendations are reasonable based upon the available evidence, but none has been validated prospectively. As such, they are based largely upon expert opinion. The following recommendations apply to individuals who have a genetic or clinical diagnosis of HNPCC or who are at increased risk for HNPCC: colonoscopy every 1–2 years beginning at age 20–25, or 10 years earlier than the youngest age of colon cancer diagnosis in the family (whichever comes first); genetic testing for HNPCC should be offered to first-degree relatives of persons with a known inherited MMR gene mutation. It should also be offered when the family mutation is not already known, but one of the first three of the modified Bethesda criteria is met.

Table 3. Lifetime risk for cancer associated with HNPCC

Types of cancer	Persons with HNPCC, %	General population, %
Colorectal	80–82	5–6
Endometrial	50–60	2–3
Gastric	13	1
Ovarian	12	1–2
Small bowel	1–4	1–2
Bladder	4	1–3
Brain	4	0.6
Kidney, renal, pelvis	3	1
Biliary tract	2	0.6

As noted above, the optimal interval for colonoscopic surveillance has not been defined in clinical trials. Some clinics recommend that colonoscopy should be performed annually in all at-risk individuals after age 40–45 since the risk of CRC increases with age. One study showed that colonoscopy on average every 3 years decreased the CRC incidence by 62% and overall mortality by 65% in 22 families with HNPCC [55]. A decision analysis estimated that colonoscopy surveillance in HNPCC family members would be associated with a gain of approximately 14 quality-adjusted life years per screened individual compared to no surveillance. This is a much greater improvement than seen with many well-accepted therapies for other diseases such as the treatment of mild hypertension. Total or subtotal colectomy with continued surveillance of the remaining rectum is recommended for patients with HNPCC who are found during surveillance to have CRC or an advanced adenoma (large, villous, or high-grade dysplasia). At present, there are no data regarding a potential role of offering primary prophylactic surgery in patients who have not yet developed an advanced lesion.

Recommendations have also been issued by other expert groups, some of which touch upon surveillance for extracolonic tumors [55]. These include: annual screening for endometrial and ovarian cancer beginning at age 25–35 years (pelvic examination and endometrial aspirate with or without transvaginal ultrasound); annual urinalysis and cytologic examination beginning at age 25; annual skin surveillance, and periodic upper endoscopy.

There have been no prospective studies to indicate how effective some of these screening programs will be, particularly those aimed at detecting gynecologic cancers. The benefits and limitations of screening were illustrated in a study involving 292 women from HNPCC or HNPCC-like families [56]. A surveillance strategy of annual or biennial (every 2 years) with either transvaginal (when available) or transabdominal ultrasound failed to detect the only 2 cases of endometrial cancer that developed during a 13-year observation period [56]. Surveillance for breast, uterine, and ovarian cancers seems warranted because of the high estimated risk. The following are recommended: breast surveillance beginning at age 25 in women with mammography beginning at age 35 is particularly important because of the markedly high risk of breast cancer; annual abdominal and pelvic ultrasound from age 25, and Papanicolaou smear every other year.

Peutz-Jeghers Syndrome

The Peutz-Jeghers syndrome (PJS) carries a 39% lifetime risk of CRC and 93% cumulative risk for the development of any type of malignancy [57]. As mentioned above, PJS has been linked to germline mutation of the *LKB1* gene. The average age of PJS diagnosis is 23–26 years, while the mean age of any cancer diagnosis is approximately 40–50 years and the mean age of CRC diagnosis is 45.8 years [57].

PJS is characterized by the presence of numerous pigmented spots on the lips and the buccal mucosa and multiple gastrointestinal hamartomatous polyps The lip pigmentation usually appears by age 2, but may fade with age. In contrast, buccal mucosal pigmentation usually persists into adulthood. Hamartomas occur most commonly in the small intestine (65–95%), but can also occur in the colon (60%), and the stomach (50%). Patients with PJS tend to develop recurrent bouts of small bowel intussusception, obstruction and bleeding, often requiring recurrent bowel resection.

Genetic testing for PJS is not yet commercially available. Because of the risk of complications related to polyps and the risk of malignancy, screening is recommended for asymptomatic first-degree relatives of patients with known PJS. None of the screening recommendations for this disease have been validated in clinical trials, but a reasonable set of recommendations includes for *first-degree relatives* upper gastrointestinal series and small bowel follow-through or an upper endoscopy and push enteroscopy at least once during the second decade of life is recommended, and for *affected individuals*, regular surveillance for polyps and their prophylactic excision is recommended once the diagnosis of PJS is established.

Upper endoscopy every other year beginning at age 10 or sooner if clinically indicated, with biopsy of all polyps to look for adenomatous change and complete removal of any polyp >1 cm has been proposed from a surveillance study [58]. A guideline issued by the British Society of Gastroenterology recommends upper gastrointestinal surveillance at 3-year intervals beginning at age 25 [59]. Colonoscopy every 3 years beginning at age 25 or sooner if clinically indicated, with biopsy of all polyps to look for adenomatous change and complete removal of any polyp >1 cm [59]. Push enteroscopy will no doubt be used increasingly to evaluate and remove polyps of the small bowel in PJS [58]. Surveillance with endoscopic ultrasound of the pancreas deserves study because of the exceptionally high risk of pancreatic cancer in PJS.

Juvenile Polyposis Coli and Familial Juvenile Polyposis

Juvenile polyposis coli (JPC) is characterized by the development of hamartomatous intestinal polyps and is associated with a 10–38% lifetime risk of CRC [60]. The median age of CRC is 34 years. The average age at which symptoms develop is 9.5 years. Patients also have a 15–21% lifetime risk of gastric and duodenal cancer [60]. The diagnosis of JPS is made when >3–10 juvenile colonic polyps are identified; or a juvenile polyp in the gastrointestinal tract outside of the colon is discovered; or any juvenile polyp is recognized in combination with family history of JPC. Germline mutations in the *SMAD4* and *BMPR1A* genes have been identified as the causative mutation in some affected families with familial juvenile polyposis (JPC) [35].

No consensus has been established for optimal screening of asymptomatic individuals at risk for FJP or for the surveillance and clinical management of patients with known juvenile polyposis.

Asymptomatic first-degree relatives of patients with JPC are at risk for juvenile polyposis and CRC and should be screened for the disease. As an example, in a kindred of 118 family members, 4 died of colonic malignancy between the ages of 30 and 55, and another 5 had juvenile polyps throughout the colon that included large lobulated polyps containing adenomatous tissue [61]. One reasonable screening strategy includes annual fecal occult blood testing and flexible sigmoidoscopy or colonoscopy every 3–5 years beginning at age 12 and continuing until approximately age 40. Symptomatic patients should be evaluated regardless of age.

A guideline issued by the British Society of Gastroenterology recommends screening of at-risk individuals with colonoscopy every 1–2 years beginning at age 15–18 (or earlier in patients who presented with symptoms) [1, 59]. Screening intervals can be extended at age 35.

In contrast, documented gene carriers or affected cases should undergo surveillance until age 70. Colonoscopic polypectomy with regular surveillance is probably adequate therapy if only a small number of polyps are present [62]. Prophylactic surgery can be considered for those [59]: with a large number of polyps; with multiple polyps that have adenomatous change and high-grade dysplasia; in which polyps cannot be removed endoscopically; in which complications (such as bleeding) are not easily controlled, and where CRC is a feature of the family history.

Upper gastrointestinal surveillance has been recommended every 1–2 years beginning at age 25 by upper endoscopy/enteroscopy or UGI with SBFT [59].

MYH Polyposis Syndrome

The discovery that biallelic mutations in the base excision repair gene, *MYH*, as described above, resulted in an increased risk of colorectal adenomas and cancer, led to the first description of an autosomal recessive colon cancer syndrome [6]. In the European population, 22–29% of individuals with >10 adenomatous polyps carried biallelic germline mutations of the *MYH* gene [6]. The precise CRC risk has not yet been ascertained, but is likely to approach the 100% level appreciated in FAP. The mean ages of colon polyps and cancer diagnosis is 46 and 49.7 years, respectively [46]. Genetic testing is now available, and analysis is focused on exons 7 and 13 of the *MYH* gene. Two specific mutations in these exons (Y165C and G382D) account for 87% of all *MYH* mutations in the Northern European population [46]. Patients who display a phenotype suggestive of AFAP but have tested negative for *APC* mutations can be offered testing for germline *MYH* mutations. It is recognized that the *MYH* syndrome has important implications for genetic counseling, as the cancer risk is limited primarily to siblings but not children. Thus far, there does not appear to be an increased risk of polyps or cancer in *MYH* heterozygote carriers.

Until official guidelines are established, it is reasonable to follow the recommendations for CRC screening in AFAP. The role of chemoprevention has not yet been studied.

Closing Remarks

There is a growing accumulation of data for the role of genetic factors in the development of CRC. A wide spectrum of genes can increase the risk of the disease when altered in the germline. The introduction of genetic testing has revolutionized the field of cancer risk assessment, and cancer prevention has become a realistic goal. The next major challenge is the identification of genetic alterations (mutations, polymorphism, imprinting loss due to epigenetic alterations) that may have low penetrance but high prevalence, as these are the genetic alterations that are likely to have an even greater impact on colon cancer risk in the population as a whole.

References

1 Jemal A, Murray T, Ward E, et al: Cancer statistics, 2005. CA Cancer J Clin 2005;55:10–30.
2 Vogelstein B, Fearon ER, Hamilton SR, et al: Genetic alterations during colorectal-tumor development. N Engl J Med 1988;319:525–532.
3 Lamlum H, Ilyas M, Rowan A, et al: The type of somatic mutation at APC in familial adenomatous polyposis is determined by the site of the germline mutation: a new facet to Knudson's 'two-hit' hypothesis. Nat Med 1999;5:1071–1075.
4 Wirtzfeld DA, Petrelli NJ, Rodriguez-Bigas MA: Hamartomatous polyposis syndromes: molecular genetics, neoplastic risk, and surveillance recommendations. Ann Surg Oncol 2001;8:319–327.
5 Lynch HT, de la CA: Hereditary colorectal cancer. N Engl J Med 2003;348:919–932.
6 Al-Tassan N, Chmiel NH, Maynard J, et al: Inherited variants of MYH associated with somatic G:C→T:A mutations in colorectal tumors. Nat Genet 2002;30:227–232.
7 Eriksson M, Brown WT, Gordon LB, et al: Recurrent de novo point mutations in lamin A cause Hutchinson-Gilford progeria syndrome. Nature 2003;423:293–298.
8 Collins FS, Green ED, Guttmacher AE, Guyer MS: A vision for the future of genomics research. Nature 2003;422:835–847.
9 Fearon ER, Vogelstein B: A genetic model for colorectal tumorigenesis. Cell 1990;61:759–767.
10 Kinzler KW, Vogelstein B: Lessons from hereditary colorectal cancer. Cell 1996;87:159–170.
11 Ionov Y, Peinado MA, Malkhosyan S, Shibata D, Perucho M: Ubiquitous somatic mutations in simple repeated sequences reveal a new mechanism for colonic carcinogenesis. Nature 1993;363:558–561.
12 Futreal PA, Coin L, Marshall M, et al: A census of human cancer genes. Nat Rev Cancer 2004;4:177–183.
13 Powell SM, Zilz N, Beazer-Barclay Y, et al: APC mutations occur early during colorectal tumorigenesis. Nature 1992;359:235–237.
14 Aaltonen LA, Peltomaki P, Leach FS, et al: Clues to the pathogenesis of familial colorectal cancer. Science 1993;260:812–816.
15 Thibodeau SN, Bren G, Schaid D: Microsatellite instability in cancer of the proximal colon. Science 1993;260:816–819.
16 Perucho M: Cancer of the microsatellite mutator phenotype. Biol Chem 1996;377:675–684.
17 Peltomaki P, Lothe RA, Aaltonen LA, et al: Microsatellite instability is associated with tumors that characterize the hereditary nonpolyposis colorectal carcinoma syndrome. Cancer Res 1993;53:5853–5855.
18 Jass JR, Do KA, Simms LA, et al: Morphology of sporadic colorectal cancer with DNA replication errors. Gut 1998;42:673–679.
19 Ajioka Y, Watanabe H, Jass JR, Yokota Y, Kobayashi M, Nishikura K: Infrequent K-ras codon 12 mutation in serrated adenomas of human colorectum. Gut 1998;42:680–684.
20 Bienz M, Clevers H: Linking colorectal cancer to Wnt signaling. Cell 2000;103:311–320.
21 Fearnhead NS, Britton MP, Bodmer WF: The ABC of APC. Hum Mol Genet 2001;10:721–733.
22 Korinek V, Barker N, Morin PJ, et al: Constitutive transcriptional activation by a β-catenin-Tcf complex in APC–/– colon carcinoma. Science 1997;275:1784–1787.
23 Van de Wetering M, Sancho E, Verweij C, et al: The β-catenin/Tcf-4 complex imposes a crypt progenitor phenotype on colorectal cancer cells. Cell 2002;111:241–250.
24 Uthoff SM, Eichenberger MR, McAuliffe TL, Hamilton CJ, Galandiuk S: Wingless-type frizzled protein receptor signaling and its putative role in human colon cancer. Mol Carcinog 2001;31:56–62.
25 Laken SJ, Petersen GM, Gruber SB, et al: Familial colorectal cancer in Ashkenazim due to a hypermutable tract in APC. Nat Genet 1997;17:79–83.
26 Drucker L, Shpilberg O, Neumann A, et al: Adenomatous polyposis coli I1307K mutation in Jewish patients with different ethnicity: prevalence and phenotype. Cancer 2000; 88:755–760.
27 Takayama T, Ohi M, Hayashi T, et al: Analysis of K-ras, APC, and β-catenin in aberrant crypt foci in sporadic adenoma, cancer, and familial adenomatous polyposis. Gastroenterology 2001;121:599–611.
28 Bourne HR, Sanders DA, McCormick F: The GTPase superfamily: conserved structure and molecular mechanism. Nature 1991; 349:117–127.
29 Pretlow TP, Brasitus TA, Fulton NC, Cheyer C, Kaplan EL: K-ras mutations in putative preneoplastic lesions in human colon. J Natl Cancer Inst 1993;85:2004–2007.
30 Kirsch DG, Kastan MB: Tumor-suppressor p53: implications for tumor development and prognosis. J Clin Oncol 1998;16:3158–3168.
31 Keino-Masu K, Masu M, Hinck L, et al: Deleted in colorectal cancer (DCC) encodes a netrin receptor. Cell 1996;87:175–185.
32 Chan SS, Zheng H, Su MW, et al: UNC-40, a *C. elegans* homolog of DCC (deleted in colorectal cancer), is required in motile cells responding to UNC-6 netrin cues. Cell 1996; 87:187–195.
33 Reiss M, Santoro V, de Jonge RR, Vellucci VF: Transfer of chromosome 18 into human head and neck squamous carcinoma cells: evidence for tumor suppression by Smad4/DPC4. Cell Growth Differ 1997;8:407–415.
34 Eppert K, Scherer SW, Ozcelik H, et al: MADR2 maps to 18q21 and encodes a TGF-β-regulated MAD-related protein that is functionally mutated in colorectal carcinoma. Cell 1996;86:543–552.
35 Fogt F, Brown CA, Badizadegan K, Zimmerman RL, Odze R: Low prevalence of loss of heterozygosity and SMAD4 mutations in sporadic and familial juvenile polyposis syndrome-associated juvenile polyps. Am J Gastroenterol 2004;99:2025–2031.
36 Howe JR, Bair JL, Sayed MG, et al: Germline mutations of the gene encoding bone morphogenetic protein receptor 1A in juvenile polyposis. Nat Genet 2001;28:184–187.
37 Hemminki A, Markie D, Tomlinson I, et al: A serine/threonine kinase gene defective in Peutz-Jeghers syndrome. Nature 1998;391: 184–187.
38 Yoo LI, Chung DC, Yuan J: LKB1 – a master tumour suppressor of the small intestine and beyond. Nat Rev Cancer 2002;2:529–535.
39 Hawley SA, Boudeau J, Reid JL, et al: Complexes between the LKB1 tumor suppressor, STRAD α/β and MO25 α/β are upstream kinases in the AMP-activated protein kinase cascade. J Biol 2003;2:28.
40 Woods A, Johnstone SR, Dickerson K, et al: LKB1 is the upstream kinase in the AMP-activated protein kinase cascade. Curr Biol 2003;13:2004–2008.
41 Popat S, Hubner R, Houlston RS: Systematic review of microsatellite instability and colorectal cancer prognosis. J Clin Oncol 2005;23:609–618.
42 Papadopoulos N, Nicolaides NC, Liu B, et al: Mutations of GTBP in genetically unstable cells. Science 1995;268:1915–1917.
43 Herman JG, Baylin SB: Gene silencing in cancer in association with promoter hypermethylation. N Engl J Med 2003;349:2042–2054.
44 Fujiwara T, Stolker JM, Watanabe T, et al: Accumulated clonal genetic alterations in familial and sporadic colorectal carcinomas with widespread instability in microsatellite sequences. Am J Pathol 1998;153:1063–1078.
45 Sieber OM, Lipton L, Crabtree M, et al: Multiple colorectal adenomas, classic adenomatous polyposis, and germ-line mutations in MYH. N Engl J Med 2003;348:791–799.
46 Sampson JR, Dolwani S, Jones S, et al: Autosomal recessive colorectal adenomatous polyposis due to inherited mutations of MYH. Lancet 2003;362:39–41.
47 Wang L, Baudhuin LM, Boardman LA, et al: MYH mutations in patients with attenuated and classic polyposis and with young-onset colorectal cancer without polyps. Gastroenterology 2004;127:9–16.

48 Croitoru ME, Cleary SP, Di NN, et al: Association between biallelic and monoallelic germline MYH gene mutations and colorectal cancer risk. J Natl Cancer Inst 2004;96:1631–1634.
49 Kambara T, Whitehall VL, Spring KJ, et al: Role of inherited defects of MYH in the development of sporadic colorectal cancer. Genes Chromosomes Cancer 2004;40:1–9.
50 Enholm S, Hienonen T, Suomalainen A, et al: Proportion and phenotype of MYH-associated colorectal neoplasia in a population-based series of Finnish colorectal cancer patients. Am J Pathol 2003;163:827–832.
51 Vasen HF, Mecklin JP, Khan PM, Lynch HT: The International Collaborative Group on Hereditary Non-Polyposis Colorectal Cancer (ICG-HNPCC). Dis Colon Rectum 1991;34:424–425.
52 Vasen HF, Watson P, Mecklin JP, Lynch HT: New clinical criteria for hereditary nonpolyposis colorectal cancer (HNPCC, Lynch syndrome) proposed by the International Collaborative Group on HNPCC. Gastroenterology 1999;116:1453–1456.
53 Rodriguez-Bigas MA, Boland CR, Hamilton SR, et al: A National Cancer Institute Workshop on Hereditary Nonpolyposis Colorectal Cancer Syndrome: meeting highlights and Bethesda guidelines. J Natl Cancer Inst 1997;89:1758–1762.
54 Umar A, Boland CR, Terdiman JP, et al: Revised Bethesda Guidelines for hereditary nonpolyposis colorectal cancer (Lynch syndrome) and microsatellite instability. J Natl Cancer Inst 2004;96:261–268.
55 Jarvinen HJ, Aarnio M, Mustonen H, et al: Controlled 15-year trial on screening for colorectal cancer in families with hereditary nonpolyposis colorectal cancer. Gastroenterology 2000;118:829–834.
56 Dove-Edwin I, Boks D, Goff S, et al: The outcome of endometrial carcinoma surveillance by ultrasound scan in women at risk of hereditary nonpolyposis colorectal carcinoma and familial colorectal carcinoma. Cancer 2002;94:1708–1712.
57 Giardiello FM, Brensinger JD, Tersmette AC, et al: Very high risk of cancer in familial Peutz-Jeghers syndrome. Gastroenterology 2000;119:1447–1453.
58 Edwards DP, Khosraviani K, Stafferton R, Phillips RK: Long-term results of polyp clearance by intraoperative enteroscopy in the Peutz-Jeghers syndrome. Dis Colon Rectum 2003;46:48–50.
59 Dunlop MG: Guidance on gastrointestinal surveillance for hereditary non-polyposis colorectal cancer, familial adenomatous polyposis, juvenile polyposis, and Peutz-Jeghers syndrome 2. Gut 2002;51(suppl 5):V21–V27.
60 Howe JR, Mitros FA, Summers RW: The risk of gastrointestinal carcinoma in familial juvenile polyposis. Ann Surg Oncol 1998;5:751–756.
61 Sharma AK, Sharma SS, Mathur P: Familial juvenile polyposis with adenomatous-carcinomatous change. J Gastroenterol Hepatol 1995;10:131–134.
62 Grotsky HW, Rickert RR, Smith WD, Newsome JF: Familial juvenile polyposis coli. A clinical and pathologic study of a large kindred. Gastroenterology 1982;82:494–501.

Review Article

Digestive Diseases

Dig Dis 2007;25:20–32
DOI: 10.1159/000099167

Preoperative Imaging Staging of Rectal Cancer

A.H. Karantanas S. Yarmenitis N. Papanikolaou N. Gourtsoyiannis

Department of Radiology, University of Crete, Heraklion, Greece

Key Words
Rectum neoplasms · Lymphatic system, rectum · Metastatic disease, rectum · MR imaging/diagnosis · Cancer staging · Rectum sonography · Rectum CT

Abstract
Carcinomas of the rectum are associated with a significant local and distant recurrence rate. Not all patients are appropriate candidates for preoperative radiation therapy. Preoperative identification of those most likely to benefit from neoadjuvant therapy is important. There is no general consensus on the role of endorectal ultrasonography, computed tomography (CT), and magnetic resonance imaging (MRI) in staging patients with rectal cancer. Although the tumor stage is an important prognostic factor, preoperative assessment is associated with prediction of the circumferential resection margin. Newer developments such as coils, sequences and gradients in MRI, evolution of multidetector CT and new contrast media, allow for an algorithm selection aiming at the best diagnostic options for patients. The present review will discuss the current role of the various imaging modalities in staging carcinomas of the rectum.

Introduction

Rectal cancer is a common malignant disease in Western countries with a high rate of mortality. Numerous improvements in the surgical, radiologic, and oncologic treatment have been made over the past two decades. Poor prognosis of rectal cancer is associated with its high risk of metastases and local recurrence.

Total mesorectal excision (TME) is defined as the resection of both the tumor and the surrounding mesorectal fat and currently is the surgical treatment of choice for rectal carcinoma. This treatment has been shown to reduce the mortality rate from 16 to 9% [1]. In addition, TME is associated with a recurrence rate of less than 10% when used as an isolated treatment option [2]. Inadequate surgical excision with microscopically infiltrated resection margins may result in a local recurrence rate of up to 83% [3]. Incomplete removal of the lateral spread of the tumor seems to be responsible for the majority of these recurrences [4]. The use of preoperative radiation therapy in patients with involvement of the mesorectal fascia at the time of diagnosis has been shown to reduce the recurrence rate from 8.2 to 2.4% at 2 years [2, 5]. The indications for preoperative radiation therapy vary between USA and Europe [6, 7]. Prerequisites for this treatment option include accurate preoperative tumor staging with regard to tumor detection, mesorectal fat infiltration, mesorectal fascia status, nodal involvement and distal metastatic disease. The contribution of imaging in

KARGER

Fax +41 61 306 12 34
E-Mail karger@karger.ch
www.karger.com

0257–2753/07/0251–0020$23.50/0

Accessible online at:
www.karger.com/ddi

A. Karantanas, MD, PhD
Department of Radiology, University Hospital
GR–711 10 Stavrakia/Heraklion (Greece)
Tel. +30 2810 392 541, Fax +30 2810 542 095
E-Mail karantanas@med.uoc.gr or apolsen@yahoo.com

rectal cancer is to classify cases on the basis of the risks of recurrence. The present review will discuss the current role of various imaging modalities, including newer developments, in staging rectal carcinoma.

T Stage

Preoperative T staging of a rectal tumor is not a simple process. Digital examination is considered unreliable [6], whereas the results of computed tomography (CT) are variable, particularly for early tumors [8]. At present, there is no widely accepted protocol on the role of diagnostic imaging in the preoperative T staging of rectal cancer. In one study, a survey in 142 departments in UK showed that only 50% of rectal cancer cases do have access for transrectal ultrasonography (TRUS) or magnetic resonance imaging (MRI) [9].

CT has been used widely for preoperative assessment of disseminated disease but its role in local staging is limited with reported accuracies ranging from 33 to 82% [10, 11]. In a recent meta-analysis of 78 studies in 4,897 patients with rectal cancer, CT showed an accuracy of 73% for T staging [12]. Multidetector technology allows for a multiplanar imaging, but there are limited prospective studies to address a newer role for CT in this respect [13]. Although spatial resolution has improved considerably with multidetector CT, its limitation remains the inherent low contrast resolution. Carcinomas of the rectum are demonstrated as focal, irregular wall thickening lesions on CT. For small tumors without any associated wall thickening, contrast enhancement in the arterial phase may be the only indicator of tumor growth [14].

TRUS is helpful in determining the depth of invasion of early-stage disease with a reported accuracy of 64–96% [15, 16]. The outermost hypoechoic layer corresponds to the muscularis propria. Carcinomas are hypoechoic, and the degree to which they disrupt and penetrate the rectal wall layers suggests the local stage. T1 tumors do not penetrate the muscularis propria and the preservation of a bright sonographic layer medial to the muscularis, represents an intact submucosa. T2 tumors penetrate the muscularis propria and so merge with it (fig. 1). T3 tumors proceed beyond the muscularis propria infiltrating the perirectal fat to a variable degree. TRUS however cannot reliably visualize the mesorectal fascia and thus cannot indicate whether the planned surgical circumferential resection margin (CRM) will be successful. Other limitations of TRUS are the operator-dependent quality of the examination and the inability to pass the probe through obstructing tumors. The proportion of early-stage disease in which local excision is the treatment of choice is only 5%. For all the above reasons, TRUS has not been adopted as the imaging modality of choice for preoperative local staging of rectal cancer.

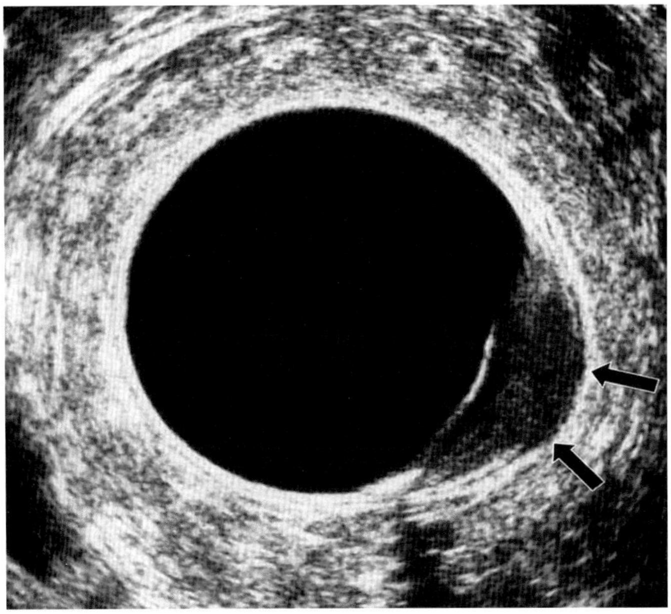

Fig. 1. TRUS in a patient with rectal carcinoma shows that the hypoechoic tumor invades the muscular wall (arrows).

The main challenge for radiological staging today is to address accurately the relationship of the tumor and the mesorectal fascia. A recent study of 686 patients undergoing TME showed that local recurrence was only 5% in those with a disease-free CRM as opposed to 22% if infiltrated [17]. MRI has been applied from its early days for staging rectal cancer, with a limited accuracy originally [18]. The development of endorectal coils improved the accuracy [19]. Further developments in phased-array coils, gradients and pulse sequences obviated the need of endorectal coils since accuracy increased up to 100% [20]. MRI with phased-array coils is able to provide detailed anatomy of the rectum and perirectal structures (fig. 2). In a study though of 76 patients, Beets-Tan et al. [21] found a moderate prediction of T stage by MRI with considerable interobserver variability (67 and 83% for two readers). In the same study, the prediction of mesorectal fascia involvement was much higher with excellent interobserver agreement, thus allowing an MRI disease-free distance of 5 and 6 mm to correspond to a histopathological disease-free margin of 1 and 2 mm, respectively

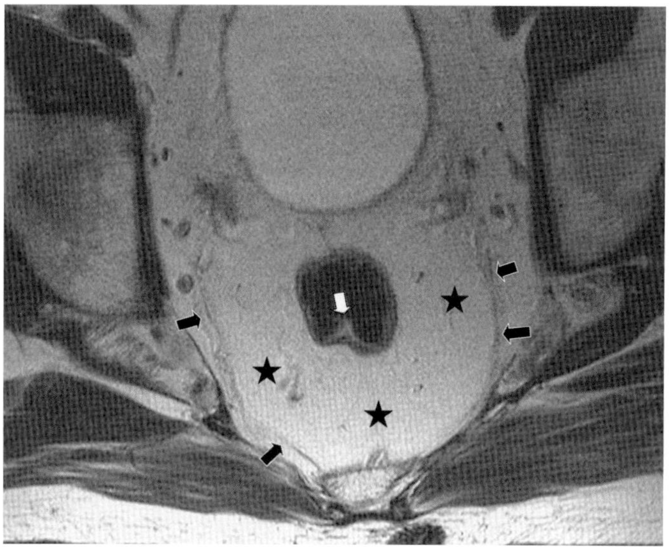

Fig. 2. Normal MRI anatomy in a 72-year-old male patient. The axial T2-w turbo spin-echo MR image shows the high signal intensity of the rectal mucosa (white arrow), the intact mesorectal fat (asterisks) and the normal appearance of the mesorectal fascia (black arrows).

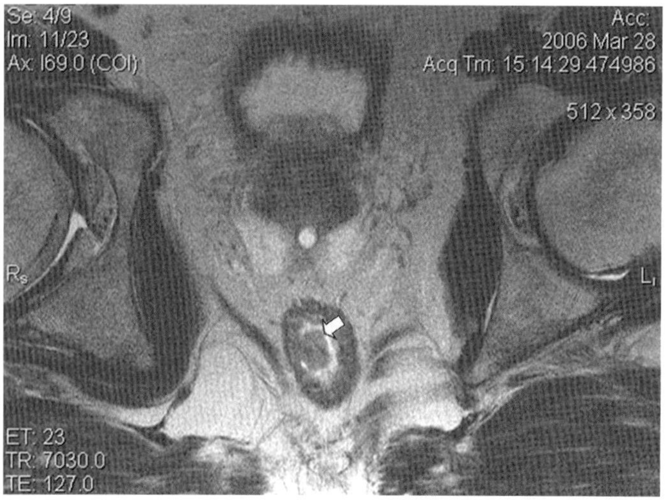

Fig. 3. Stage T1 rectal carcinoma. The axial T2-w turbo spin-echo MR image shows the small intraluminal polypoid lesion (arrow) with no disruption of the muscular layer.

[21]. One study in 98 rectal cancer patients showed 92% agreement between MR images and histologic findings for prediction of the CRM [22]. Another study in 43 patients not only confirmed a high accuracy (95%) for prediction of CRM but in addition proved in cadavers that the thin linear structure seen on MRI indeed corresponds to the mesorectal fascia (fig. 2) [23]. Therefore, although the accuracy of MRI in local staging remains controversial, its efficiency in estimating the carcinoma infiltration of the mesorectal fascia is widely accepted. The differentiation between stage T2 and T3 tumors will not affect or modify the overall preoperative or operative management of the patients. The clinically relevant benefit of MRI is the assessment of the distance from the tumor to the CRM which will predict local recurrence [17, 24].

An optimized MRI technique employed should include pelvic phased-array coils, sagittal T2-w turbo spin-echo sequences through the pelvis to detect the tumor, and then high-resolution T2-w examinations perpendicular to the tumor's long axis and in coronal plane, using FOV of 16–18 cm, thin sections of 3–4 mm and high matrix of up to 512 × 512. Axial T1-w images of the entire pelvis are always used for detecting lymphadenopathy. Routine use of intravenous contrast does not seem to increase accuracy [25]. On T2-w images, carcinomas appear as wall lesions exhibiting signal intensity slightly higher than the muscularis propria. High signal intensity of the tumor on T2-w images suggests the presence of mucinous carcinoma which has a worse prognosis compared to the non-mucinous one [26]. The outermost margin of the muscularis propria will remain intact with stage T2 tumors or less (fig. 3). Differentiation between T2 and T3 tumors may be difficult with MRI and overstaging is often caused by perirectal desmoplastic reactions which do not contain tumor cells [20, 21].

For T3 tumors with disease-free circumferential margins, it was shown that >5 mm spread of tumor beyond the bowel wall predicts a significantly poorer survival than <5 mm spread (fig. 4–6) [27]. A possible limitation of MRI, not addressed so far, is the converging of the muscularis propria and the mesorectal fascia anteriorly and towards the anal canal where a very early T3 lesion can still theoretically infiltrate the mesorectal fascia [28]. Another issue not addressed yet in the literature is the ability of MRI to depict the mesorectal fascia in all patients, regardless of the level of the tumor and the body weight. Vascular invasion of a rectal carcinoma is associated with an increased rate of local recurrence [29, 30]. The presence of a tubular structure in proximity to a T3 rectal tumor or to nodules with irregular margins probably represents vascular invasion [22, 31] (fig. 6).

Stage T4 tumors are diagnosed by depicting infiltration into an adjacent organ (fig. 7). For locally advanced carcinoma of the rectum, MRI is superior to CT for estimating invasion of surrounding organs, pelvic wall and bone marrow [32, 33]. In patients with advanced disease, a baseline MRI before radiotherapy should be performed because it is not easy to differentiate post-radiation fibrosis from viable tumor within fibrosis [34].

N Stage

Evaluation of lymph node metastatic involvement is a difficult task for radiologists. Lymph node neoplastic infiltration has been assessed for a long time by using morphological criteria such as the size and shape. A node measuring >8 mm in the short axis is probably malignant [35]. Enlarged nodes however may be benign and reactive whereas small nodes may be infiltrated. For rectal cancer in particular, over half of the metastatic nodes secondary to rectal cancer are <5 mm and are located within 3 cm of the primary tumor [36, 37]. In a large trial, lymph node metastatic disease was shown to predict local recurrence [2]. In this study, patients with stage III had a 10- and 3-fold higher risk for local recurrence than did those with stage I and II, respectively. Recent studies with TME as the treatment of choice showed that there is no association of nodal involvement and rate of local recurrence [12, 38, 39]. Therefore, nodal involvement might be clinically irrelevant if an adequate disease-free margin exists. TME however does not remove the internal iliac nodes. Lower rectal cancer is associated with internal iliac nodes involvement in 28%, and in 6% of cases those lateral nodes seem to be the only lymph nodes involved [40]. MRI depiction of the nodes lateral to mesorectal fascia is clinically important since if detected they must be included in the radiation field. Extended removal is not indicated as it results in significant urinary and sexual dysfunction.

There is a wide variation in accuracy for metastatic nodal detection with TRUS (62–87%), CT (22–73%) and MRI (39–95%) [12, 15, 41–46]. TRUS applies the criteria of lack of ovoid morphology and central echogenic nidus, but its inherently limited field of view is a major limitation. CT is based on size alone and therefore is not reliable. High-resolution MRI with the inherent contrast between fat and lesions predicts nodal involvement most accurately when the morphological features, such as a spiculated or indistinct border and a mottled heterogeneous appearance, are used rather than the size alone [35, 47] (fig. 4–6). The use of size therefore as a criterion for determining nodal involvement in rectal cancer is not recommended. Invisible lymph nodes preoperatively are a highly specific MRI indication of disease-free nodal status [35]. The rate

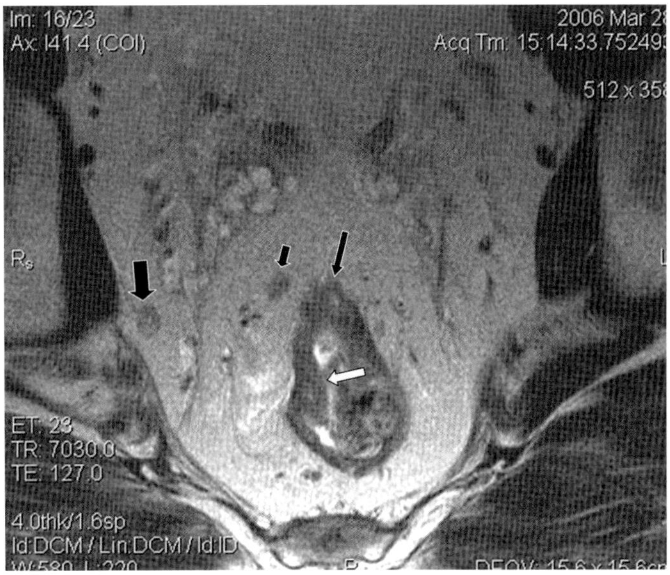

Fig. 4. Stage T3 rectal carcinoma without involvement of the mesorectal fascia. The axial T2-w turbo spin-echo MR image shows a neoplastic rectal lesion with intraluminal component (white arrow) which disrupts the integrity of the muscular layer and invades the surrounding mesorectal fat anteriorly (black arrow). A small node in the mesorectal fat (small arrow) has irregular margins and histologically was invaded by tumor cells. A node lateral to the mesorectal fascia (thick arrow) has sharp margins and presumably is benign (on follow-up studies there was no change of size).

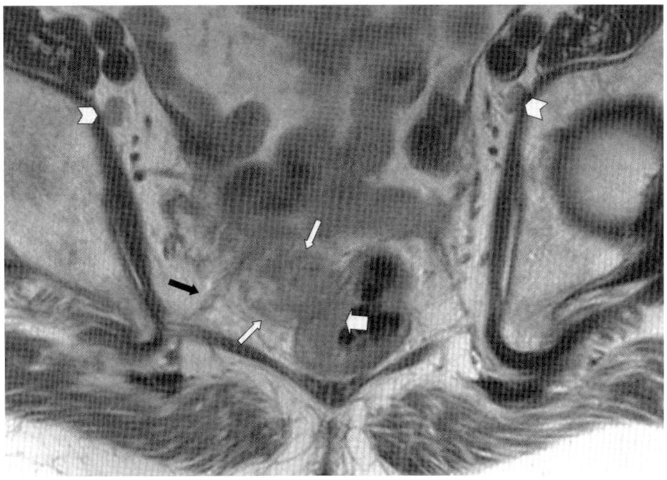

Fig. 5. Rectal cancer with involved mesorectal resection plane in a 71-year-old man. Axial T2-w turbo spin-echo MR image shows a bulky stage T3 tumor in the right lateral rectal wall (white thick arrow) extending to perirectal fat (white arrows) in close proximity to the mesorectal fascia which is thickened (black arrow). CRM was predicted to be 0 mm. Well-marginated iliac lymph nodes (arrowheads) are probably non-malignant.

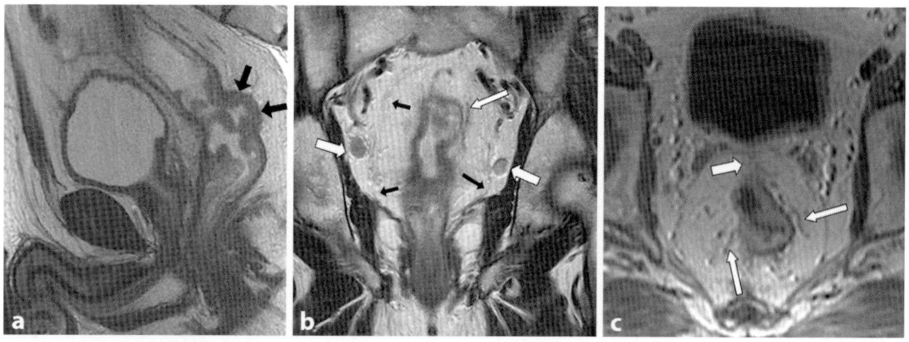

6

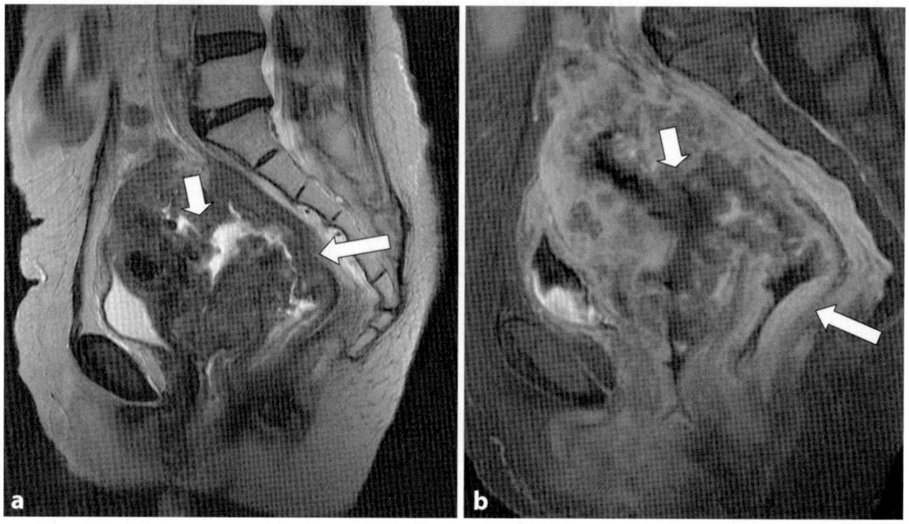

7

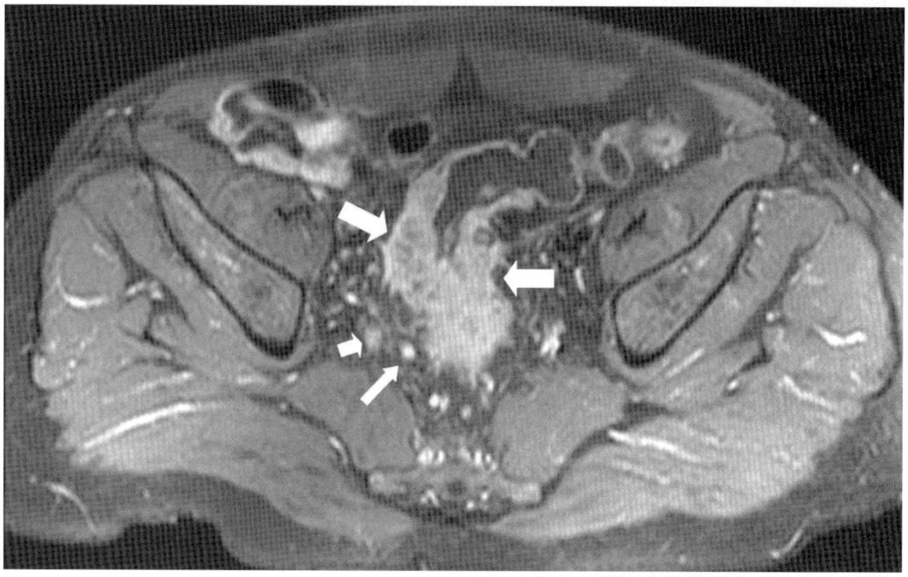

8

Fig. 6. T3 rectal carcinoma in a 53-year-old male patient. **a** Sagittal T2-w MR image shows the neoplastic wall thickening (arrows). **b** Coronal T2-w MR image shows lymph nodes (white arrows) lateral to the mesorectal fascia (black arrows) with sharp margins suggesting reactive status. A tubular structure (long white arrow) represents vascular invasion. **c** Axial contrast-enhanced T1-w MR image shows anterior extension of the tumor, in close proximity to the mesorectal fascia (short arrow). Vascular invasion is demonstrated with the presence of tubular structures (long arrows).

Fig. 7. Stage T4 rectal cancer. Sagittal T2-w (**a**) and contrast-enhanced T1-w (**b**) MR images show a mucinous rectal carcinoma (long arrow) extended anteriorly to invade the posterior myometrium (short arrow).

Fig. 8. Stage T3 rectal cancer. The axial contrast-enhanced fat-suppressed T1-w MR image shows the intense enhancement of the tumor (thick arrows), and two nodes in the perirectal fat with intense (thin arrow) and moderate (short arrow) enhancement, of unclear predictive value.

and degree of nodal enhancement has not been yet addressed in the literature to provide any additional information (fig. 8). The recent development of lymph node-specific contrast agents will aid in detecting tumorous involvement in normal-sized nodes [48]. A node with mixed or increased signal intensity will be probably malignant, whereas a node with central or uniform low signal intensity at T2*-w MR images non-malignant.

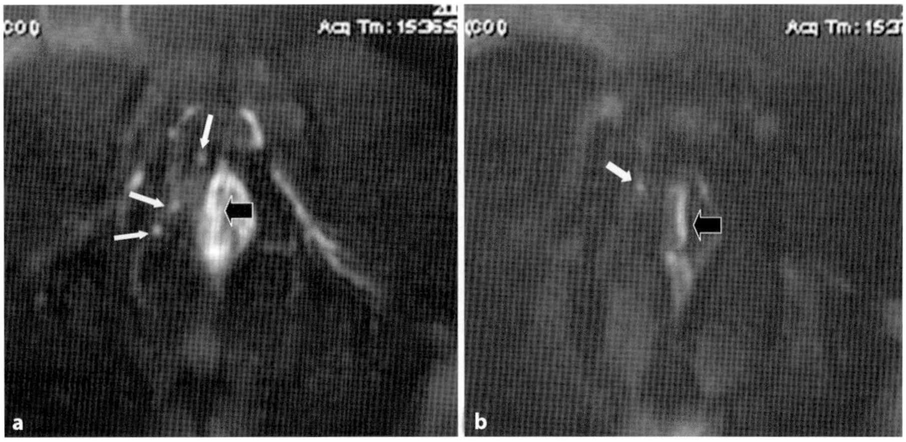

Fig. 9. Diffusion-weighted imaging. **a** Non-diffusion-weighted (b = 0) image shows high signal intensity of the tumor (black arrow) and 3 nodes in the perirectal fat (white arrows). **b** On diffusion-weighted image (b = 1,000), only one of the nodes (white arrow) and the tumor (black arrow) exhibit high signal intensity, due to restricted diffusion.

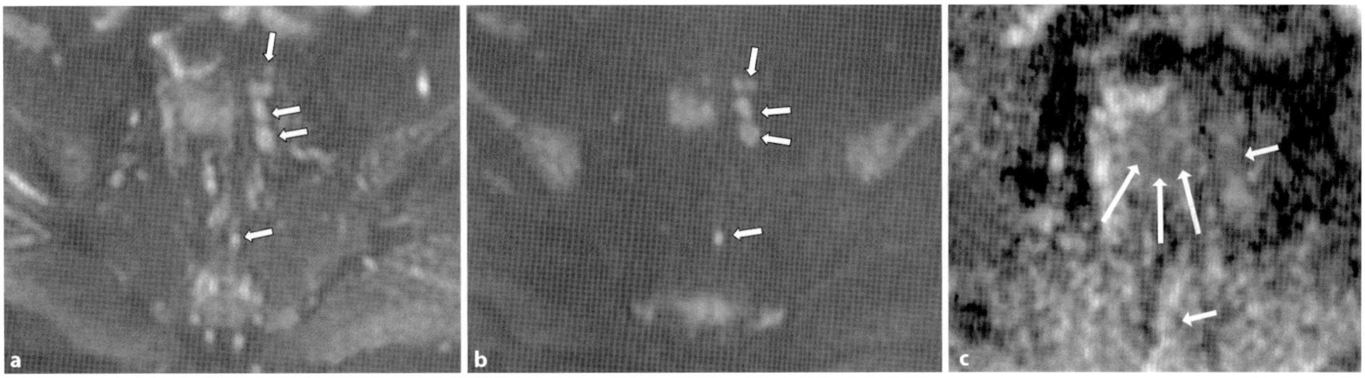

Fig. 10. Diffusion-weighted imaging. **a** On the non-diffusion-weighted image (b = 0), multiple peritumoral lymph nodes and a small-sized distant one are shown (arrows). **b, c** On diffusion-weighted image (b = 1,000) the lymph nodes maintain high signal intensity, whereas in the ADC map (**c**) only the middle of the group and the small distant (small arrows) possess restricted diffusion together with the tumor (large arrows).

Recently, the application of diffusion-weighted imaging, a relatively old idea that proved to be very successful in detecting acute brain ischemia, has shown to be feasible in abdominal areas [49]. According to this technique, it is possible to detect early changes in the architecture of tissue and differentiate malignant from benign lesions on the basis of hypercellularity commonly found in malignancies. The signal in diffusion-weighted images strongly depends on the diffusion of water molecules, mainly located in the extracellular space. Whenever there is an alteration in the size of the extracellular space, the diffusion pattern is directly affected. It has been shown that increased cellularity causes a reduction in size of the extracellular space, therefore diffusion is restricted in such a case and the corresponding quantitative parameter, namely the apparent diffusion coefficient (ADC) is reduced. On the contrary, whenever there is an increase in the size of extracellular space due to increased water content, there is an elevation of the ADC. In this content, malignant lymph nodes might be possible to be differentiated from inflammatory due to lower ADC values that may exhibit (fig. 9, 10). In addition, it has been shown that ADC measurements may also help in assessing post-radiation fibrosis [50].

M Stage

Distant metastatic disease in patients with rectal carcinoma is most commonly located in the liver. Studies have shown that patients who die of cancer are found at autopsy to have liver metastases with a frequency of 25–

50%. In patients with colorectal cancer, 40% on average develop liver metastases [51]. Hepatic metastatic disease is associated with poor prognosis.

The liver is a unique organ with regard to its dual blood supply pattern (arterial and portal) and its vulnerability to metastatic disease. It is reported that hepatic metastases undergo a complex process regarding the development of their vasculature and particularly the relative contribution of the portal vein and the hepatic artery in the blood supply [52–56]. Thus, tumor vascularity is a continuously changing phenomenon. In the very early phase, the neoplastic cells are expected to receive nourishment by diffusion from surrounding vessels. This happens until the metastatic focus reaches a size of 150–200 mm [57]. As tumor grows, angiogenesis occurs with vessels arising either from arterial or portal components. The portal contribution seems to decline as the tumor exceeds 2 mm in size and the arterial role predominates [54]. An additional characteristic of importance is that metastases, unlike the normal liver parenchyma, lack Kupffer cells. In general, most metastases from rectal carcinoma are hypovascular receiving blood supply from the hepatic artery whereas normal liver parenchyma receives 60–70% of its blood supply from the portal vein.

The progress that has been achieved in the past two decades in medical imaging has offered the ability to visualize small-sized metastatic lesions (<1 cm) achieving a sensitivity of as high as 90% [58]. Unfortunately, the ability of an imaging modality to depict a parenchymal focal lesion does not depend solely on size. Other factors relative to the biological stage of the metastatic process (i.e. tumor vascularity) seem to influence the depiction ability of modern imaging modalities [59, 60]. Subsequently, neither of the imaging tests in their conventional versions could provide negative predictive values greater than 70% [61]. Newer developments are currently being assessed clinically including multidetector CT scanners, high-field MR scanners with fast MR sequences and phased-array coils, use of superparamagnetic or hepatocyte-specific MR contrast agents and ultrasound contrast agents, and PET-CT.

Ultrasonography

Ultrasonography (US) is currently the most commonly applied imaging modality for assessing hepatic metastases. Baseline gray-scale US is the first-line technique exhibiting a sensitivity ranging from 40 to 80% depending on the diameter of the lesions and the experience of the sonologist [62].

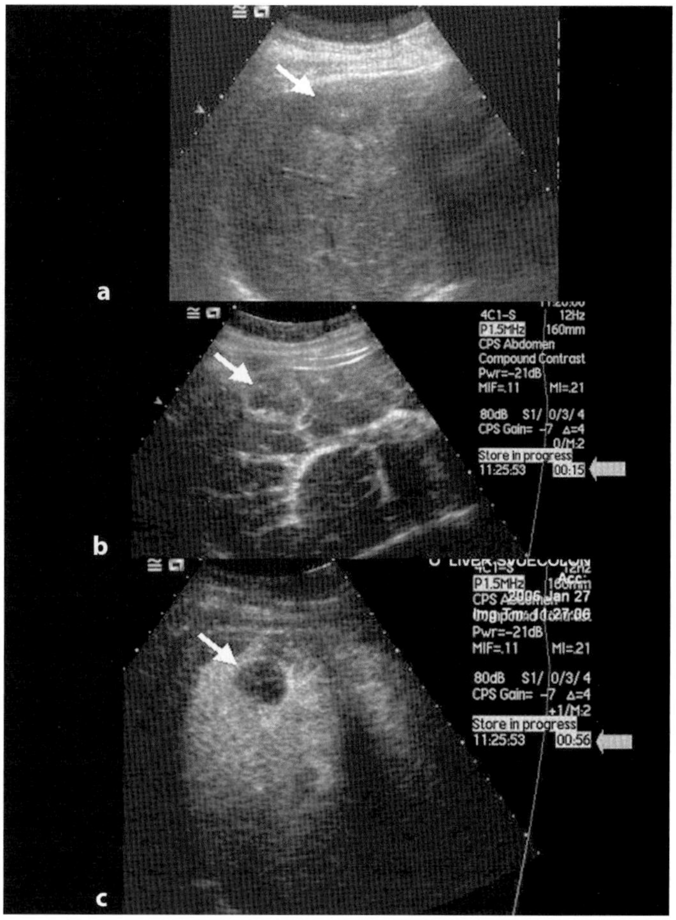

Fig. 11. Ultrasound liver scan of a 64-year-old female with rectosigmoid colon adenocarcinoma and a metastatic lesion located at segment V of the liver parenchyma (arrows). **a** At baseline scan the lesion is hyporeflective with some degree of echogenic center. **b** At the arterial phase there is a ring-like peripheral enhancement with the rest of the lesion remaining hypovascular. **c** At the sinusoidal phase, the metastasis remains hypovascular and is clearly depicted from the surrounding enhanced normal parenchyma. Thick arrows in **b** and **c** denote time counter in seconds after intravenous contrast injection.

The introduction of US contrast agents and the advances in ultrasound apparatuses, able to detect these agents in real time, have improved the overall accuracy of baseline US in liver metastatic disease, both for detection and monitoring the effect of therapy [63–67]. There are no reports yet to describe the performance of the newer systems exclusively on patients with colorectal cancer liver metastases. A recent work from Quaia et al. [68] compared prospectively contrast-enhanced ultrasound versus baseline ultrasound and contrast-enhanced spiral CT in metastatic disease of the liver in general. This is the

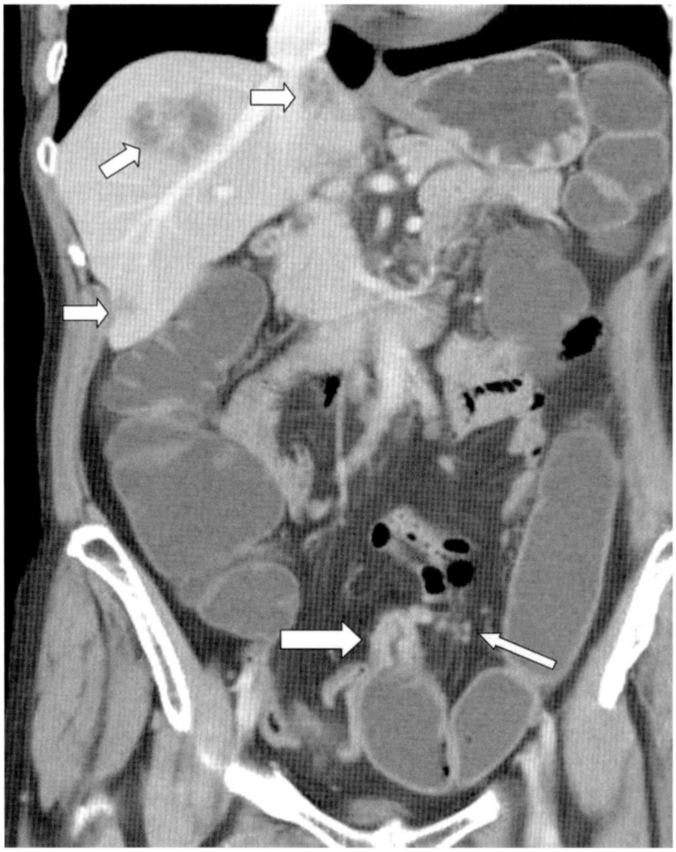

Fig. 12. The coronal reconstruction of a multidetector CT study (portal phase) in a patient with rectosigmoid carcinoma shows the wall thickening of the tumor (arrow), multiple small nodes (thin arrow) and multiple liver metastases (short arrows).

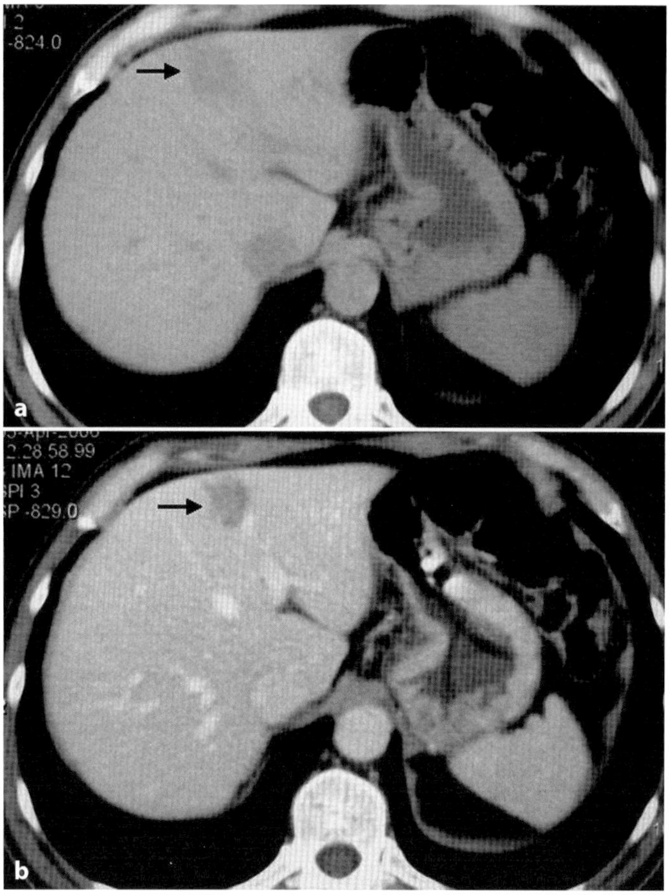

Fig. 13. CT scan of the liver of a 77-year-old male with rectal cancer and a metastasis between segments VIII and IVa (black arrows). **a** At pre-contrast scan the lesion is hypoattenuating and poorly defined. **b** At late portal venous phase the lesion is clearly demonstrated as a hypovascularized focus surrounded by the normally enhanced liver parenchyma.

only study on the topic and contrast-enhanced US was found to show an 83% sensitivity, 84% specificity and a high accuracy as shown by a 0.929 ROC under the curve analysis. Sonographically, after the intravenous contrast administration, the colorectal hepatic metastases present a hypovascular pattern as early as the arterial phase with a perilesional enhancing rim. They remain hyporeflective at the portal phase compared to the surrounding liver parenchyma (fig. 11). The gold-standard reference in US fields is the intraoperative examination of the liver which is widely accepted to approach a 100% sensitivity in detecting metastatic disease.

Computed Tomography

CT is generally considered the primary imaging modality for diagnosis and preoperative staging in patients suffering from primary cancers of the abdomen. It provides wide availability and simultaneous evaluation of primary cancer, as well as metastatic disease. However, the reported sensitivity of single-detector row helical CT for the detection of hepatic metastases, as compared with other recently established liver imaging modalities, remains unsatisfactory [69–71]. Furthermore, the accurate characterization of small hepatic metastases with helical CT alone is often difficult, since small hepatic cysts are the most frequently encountered cause of low attenuation focal lesions on CT [72]. A recent meta-analysis comparing imaging modalities in colorectal liver metastasis showed that contrast-enhanced CT shows sensitivity ranging from 70 to 85%, or even lower for lesions <1 cm in diameter [73]. Higher sensitivity (87.1%) has been reported for CT arterial portography, but this technique,

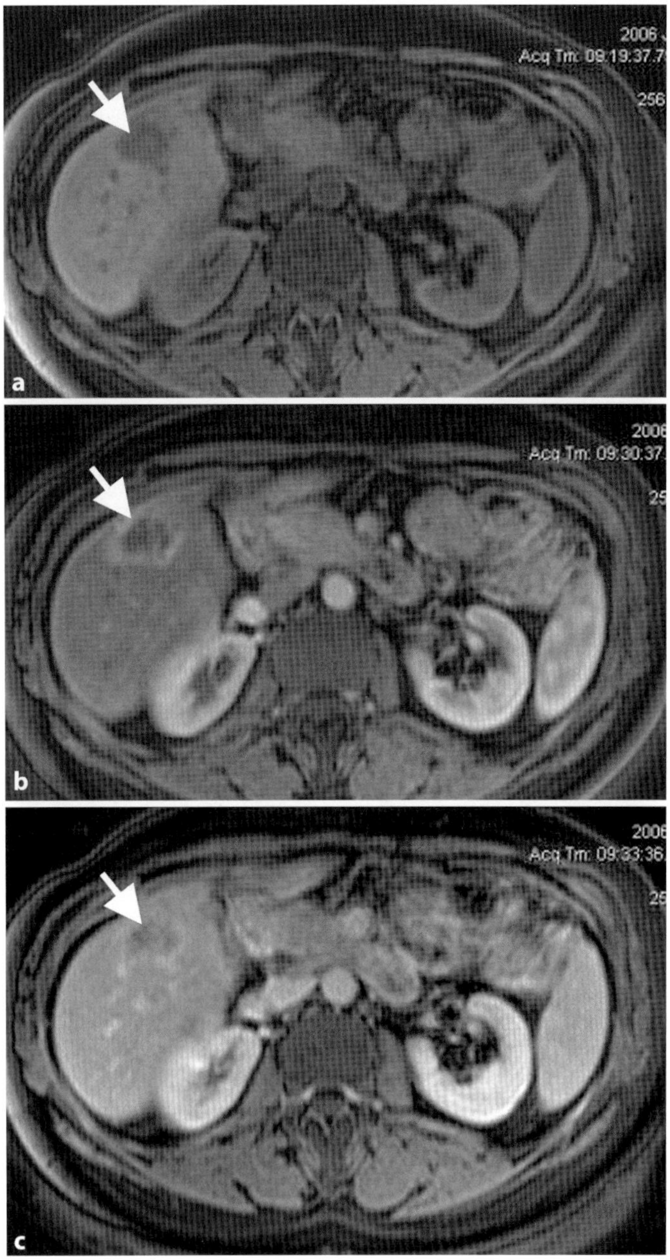

Fig. 14. MRI scan of the same patient as in figure 11. **a** T1-w transverse scan with fat suppression. The hepatic metastasis at segment V is hypointense (arrow). **b** Post-contrast transverse scan at arterial phase shows a hyperintense ring-like enhancement of the lesion (arrow), which is centrally hypovascular. **c** Post-contrast transverse scan at portal venous phase illustrates washout of the peripheral enhancement of the metastasis (arrow), which remains hypovascular compared to the rest of the normally enhanced liver parenchyma.

although still favored by some institutions, relies on interventional angiographic procedures and is usually related to high rates of false-positive diagnoses [74]. Metastatic lesions in CT may be hypodense or isodense to the normal parenchyma. Contrast-enhanced CT scanning is performed as a standard portal venous (hepatic) phase study utilizing a minimum 42-gram iodine load modified according to patient weight. The lesions appear hypodense for reasons discussed previously (fig. 12, 13). In patients who are potential surgical candidates, an additional arterial-phase CT series is acquired for accurate arterial and portal branches mapping.

Magnetic Resonance Imaging

Colorectal hepatic metastases most commonly appear as lesions that are moderately hyperintense on T2-w images and hypointense on T1-w images. Gadolinium-based intravenous contrast agents can improve the sensitivity of MRI in detecting metastases. During dynamically enhanced scanning, metastases may be of increased signal during the arterial phase and decreased signal in the portal phase, but as a general rule they are usually hypovascular in arterial phase. They may also show peripheral washout with the periphery of the metastasis being of lower signal than the center and adjacent liver. On delayed scanning, metastases may have increased signal [75, 76] (fig. 14). The absence of Kupffer cells in the metastatic foci is exploited by MRI using iron oxides. This superparamagnetic agent is taken up in Kupffer cells resulting in a lower signal in normal liver but no change in the signal of the metastasis on T2-w images, thus increasing overall conspicuity (fig. 15).

In a recent study that compares 16-row multidetector CT versus SPIO-enhanced MRI, the sensitivity was 80 and 94.5%, respectively ($p < 0.05$) [77]. In the aforementioned meta-analysis study, SPIO-enhanced MRI was the most accurate modality ($p < 0.001$) [73].

Diffusion-weighted imaging has been proposed as an alternative source of contrast to differentiate more accurately malignant from benign focal liver lesions [48]. As explained previously, malignant lesions present with increased cellularity therefore exhibit restricted diffusion, in contrast to benign lesions where increased extracellular space is resulting in free diffusion. In case of colorectal metastasis, diffusion-weighted images show a characteristic imaging pattern of a bright focal area that corresponds most probably to necrosis surrounded by a high intensity rim that reflects an area with restricted diffusion (fig. 16).

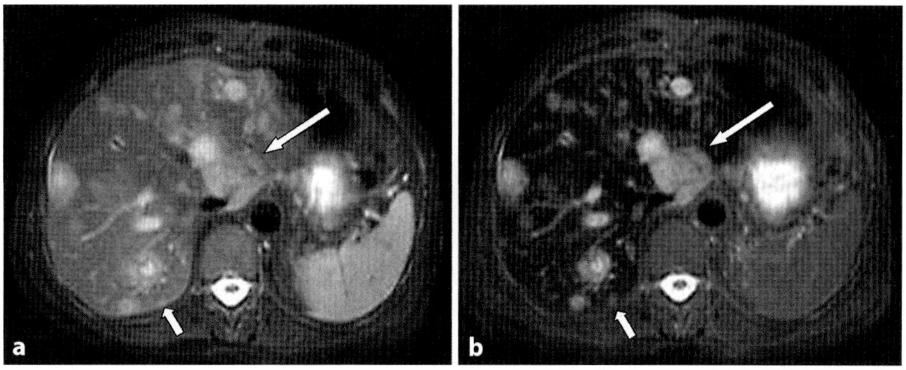

15

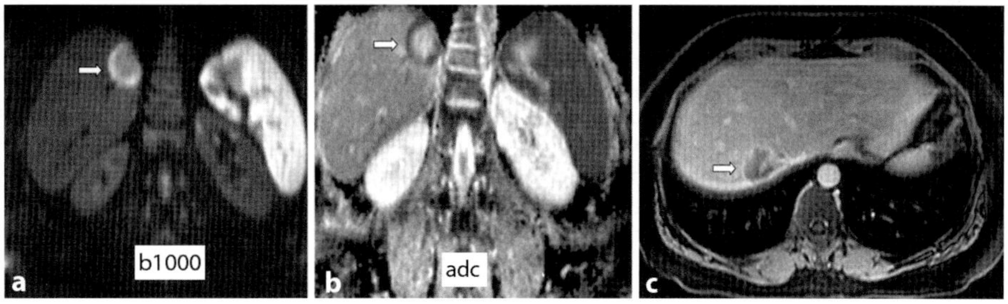

16

Fig. 15. Patient with rectal cancer and known metastatic foci in the liver. **a** The axial fat-suppressed T2-w GRASE MR image shows multiple lesions exhibiting high signal intensity (arrows). **b** After administration of superparamagnetic contrast, there is decreased signal of the liver, spleen and bone marrow. There is increased conspicuity for depicting both the large (arrow) and the small (small arrow) lesions.
Fig. 16. Liver metastatic disease. **a** The diffusion-weighted coronal image demonstrates a focal lesion with a hyperintense rim (arrow) and a low intensity central area. **b** The same lesion on the ADC map exhibits a low ADC value in the peripheral rim (arrow) and a high ADC value in the central area. **c** The post-gadolinium portal phase T1-w axial MR image shows the same lesion with peripheral enhancement characteristic of colorectal metastasis.

Positron Emission Tomography

The role of positron emission tomography (PET) or PET/CT is currently limited to assessing hepatic metastatic disease and, although sensitive, it should be used mainly as an additional imaging modality for detection of extrahepatic disease [73]. False-positive results occur secondary to inflammatory of granulomatous lesions and false-negative in cases with small tumors. PET/CT is widely accepted as a highly sensitive and specific technique in assessing local recurrence.

Detecting the Occult Colorectal Liver Metastases

Major efforts have been made thus far to establish an efficient diagnostic approach, in order to achieve the earliest possible detection of liver metastatic disease. For several years, interest has been focused on investigating the hemodynamic changes provoked by the presence of secondary neoplastic lesions of the liver. The two major fields of those studies include dynamic scintigraphic examinations and more recently color Doppler US. The former is systematically described in the works of Leveson et al. [78, 79]; the latter is extensively presented in the studies published by Leen et al. [80]. Although the concept of hemodynamic changes due to the presence of hepatic metastases was confirmed experimentally, reproducibility of these techniques was not universally proven [81, 82]. Hence the issue of occult hepatic metastases detection is still a major challenge that remains under investigation in the field of ongoing research.

Conclusions

With the newer treatment options in rectal cancer, such as preoperative radiation, preoperative chemotherapy and TME, there is an increased demand for accurate depiction by imaging the high-risk patients for local recurrence. For superficial tumors which are treated with surgery alone, TRUS is able to assess the muscular involvement. For the vast majority of rectal carcinomas, MRI will detect accurately the mesorectal fascia and the CRM. MRI is superior to CT for assessing invasion of the surrounding organs and structures. Nodal disease remains a difficult radiological diagnosis, although nodes as small as 2–3 mm can now be depicted with high-resolution MR images. For hepatic metastatic disease, the highest sensitivity (95–99%) is provided with intraoperative US, superparamagnetic iron oxide (SPIO) or gadobenate dimeglumine (Gd-BOPTA)-enhanced MRI and contrast-enhanced CT during arterial portography. The choice between portal phase helical CT performed with >45 g of iodine and MRI with a gadolinium-based contrast agent or SPIO should depend on availability and expertise and not on literature-based diagnostic accuracy alone. The contrast-enhanced ultrasound technique is the fastest emerging imaging approach, but more clinical series are expected to define its exact role. The role of multidetector CT has to be set, but for distant metastatic disease it remains the first option. Further studies should address the establishment of preoperative MRI as a useful clinical tool, the role of diffusion and perfusion imaging for preoperative staging of the primary tumor, the role of newer contrast media for detecting metastatic nodal disease and the relative accuracy of US, MRI and multidetector CT for distant metastatic disease.

References

1 Goh V, Halligan S, Bartram CI: Local radiological staging of rectal cancer. Clin Radiol 2004;59:215–226.
2 Kapiteijn E, Marijnen CA, Nagtegaal ID, et al: Preoperative radiotherapy combined with total mesorectal excision for resectable rectal cancer. N Engl J Med 2001;345:638–646.
3 Quirke P, Durdey P, Dixon MF, Williams NS: Local recurrence of rectal adenocarcinoma due to inadequate surgical resection: histopathological study of lateral tumor spread and surgical excision. Lancet 1986;ii:996–999.
4 Adam IJ, Mohamdee MO, Martin IG, et al: Role of circumferential margin involvement in the local recurrence of rectal cancer. Lancet 1994;344:707–711.
5 Beets-Tan RG, Beets GL: Rectal cancer: review with emphasis on MRI. Radiology 2004;232:335–346.
6 NIH Consensus Conference: Adjuvant therapy for patients with colon and rectal cancer. JAMA 1990;264:1444–1450.
7 Swedish Rectal Cancer Trial Investigators: Improved survival with preoperative radiotherapy in resectable rectal cancer. N Engl J Med 1997;336:980–987.
8 Nicholls RJ, Mason AY, Morson BC, et al: The clinical staging of rectal cancer. Br J Surg 1982;69:404–409.
9 Taylor A, Sheridan M, McGee S, Halligan S: Preoperative staging of rectal cancer by MRI; results of a UK survey. Clin Radiol 2005;60: 579–586.
10 Thompson WM, Halvorsen RA, Foster WL, et al: Preoperative and postoperative staging of rectosigmoid carcinoma. AJR Am J Roentgenol 1986;146:703–710.
11 Shank B, Dershaw DD, Caravelli J, et al: A prospective study of preoperative computed tomography staging of patients with biopsy proven rectal carcinoma. Dis Colon Rectum 1990;33:285–290.
12 Kwok H, Bissett IP, Hill GL: Preoperative staging of rectal cancer. Int J Colorectal Dis 2000;15:9–20.
13 Filippone A, Ambrosini R, Fuschi M, et al: Preoperative T and N staging of colorectal cancer: accuracy of contrast-enhanced multi-detector row CT colonography – initial experience. Radiology 2004;231:83–90.
14 Hundt W, Braunschweig R, Reiser M: Evaluation of spiral CT in staging of colon and rectum carcinoma. Eur Radiol 1999;9:78–84.
15 Rifkin MD, Ehrlich SM, Marks G: Staging of rectal carcinoma: prospective comparison of endorectal US and CT. Radiology 1989;170: 319–322.
16 Hunerbein M. Endorectal ultrasound in rectal cancer: Colorectal Dis 2003;5:402–405.
17 Wibe A, Rendedall PR, Svensson E, et al: Prognostic significance of the circumferential resection margin following total mesorectal excision for cancer. Br J Surg 2002;89: 327–334.
18 Butch RJ, Stark DD, Wittenberg J, et al: Staging rectal cancer by MR and CT. AJR Am J Roentgenol 1986;146:1155–1160.
19 Schnall M, Furth EE, Rosato E, Kressel HY: Rectal tumour stage: correlation of endorectal MRI and pathologic findings. Radiology 1994;190:709–714.
20 Brown G, Richards CJ, Newcombe RG, et al: Rectal carcinoma: thin section MRI for staging in 28 patients. Radiology 1999;211:215–222.
21 Beets-Tan RGH, Beets GL, Vliegen RFA, et al: Accuracy of magnetic resonance imaging in prediction of tumour-free resection margin in rectal cancer surgery. Lancet 2001;357: 497–504.
22 Brown G, Radcliffe AG, Newcombe RG, Dallimore NS, Bourne MW, Williams GT: Preoperative assessment of prognostic factors in rectal cancer using high-resolution magnetic resonance imaging. Br J Surg 2003;90: 355–364.
23 Bissett IP, Fernando CC, Hough DM, et al: Identification of the fascia propria by magnetic resonance imaging and its relevance to preoperative assessment of rectal cancer. Dis Colon Rectum 2001;44:259–265.
24 Nagtegaal ID, Marijnen CA, Kranenbarg EK, van de Velde CJ, van Krieken JH: Circumferential margin involvement is still an important predictor of local recurrence in rectal carcinoma: not one millimeter but two millimeters is the limit. Am J Surg Pathol 2002;26:350–357.
25 Vliegen RFA, Beets GL, von Meyenfeldt MF, et al: Rectal cancer: MRI in local staging-is gadolinium-based contrast material helpful? Radiology 2005;234:179–188.
26 Hussain SM, Outwater EK, Siegelman ES: Mucinous versus nonmucinous rectal carcinomas: differentiation with MRI. Radiology 1999;213:79–85.
27 Merkel S, Mansmann U, Siassi M, Papadopoulos T, Hohenberger W, Hermanek P: The prognostic inhomogeneity in pT3 rectal carcinomas. Int J Colorectal Dis 2001;16:298–304.
28 Brown H: Thin section MRI in multidisciplinary pre-operative decision making for patients with rectal cancer. Br J Radiol 2005; 78:S117–S127.
29 Talbot IC, Ritchie S, Leighton MH, Hughes AO, Bussey HJ, Morson BC: The clinical significance of invasion of veins by rectal cancer. Br J Surg 1980;67:439–442.
30 Ross A, Rusnak C, Weinerman B, Kuechler P, Hayashi A, Maclachlan G, et al: Recurrence and survival after surgical management of rectal cancer. Am J Surg 1999;177: 392–395.
31 Oh YT, Kim MJ, Lim JS, et al: Assessment of the prognostic factors for a local recurrence of rectal cancer: the utility of preoperative MRI. Korean J Radiol 2005;6:8–16.
32 Beets-Tan RG, Beets GL, Borstlap AC, et al: Preoperative assessment of local tumor extent in advanced rectal cancer: CT or high-resolution MRI? Abdom Imaging 2000;25: 533–541.
33 Blomqvist L, Holm T, Nyren S, Svanstrom R, Ulvskog Y, Iselius L: MRI and computed tomography in patients with rectal tumors clinically judged as locally advanced. Clin Radiol 2002;57:211–218.
34 Kahn H, Alexander A, Rakinic J, et al: Preoperative staging of irradiated rectal cancers using digital rectal examination, computed tomography, endorectal ultrasound, and magnetic resonance imaging does not accurately predict T0, N0 pathology. Dis Colon Rectum 1997;40:140–144.
35 Kim JH, Beets GL, Kim MJ, Kessels AG, Beets-Tan RG: High-resolution MRI for nodal staging in rectal cancer: are there any criteria in addition to the size? Eur J Radiol 2004;52:78–83.
36 Dworak O: Number and size of lymph nodes and node metastases in rectal carcinomas. Surg Endosc 1989;3:96–99.

37 Monig SP, Baldus SE, Zirbes TK, et al: Lymph node size and metastatic infiltration in colon cancer. Ann Surg Oncol 1999;6:579–581.
38 Heald RJ, Ryall RD: Recurrence and survival after total mesorectal excision for rectal cancer. Lancet 1986;i:1479–1482.
39 De Haas-Kock DF, Baeten CG, Jager JJ, et al: Prognostic significance of radial margins of clearance in rectal cancer. Br J Surg 1996;83: 781–785.
40 Moriya Y, Sugihara K, Akasu T, Fujita S: Importance of extended lymphadenectomy with lateral node dissection for advanced lower rectal cancer. World J Surg 1997;21: 728–732.
41 Katsura Y, Yamada K, Ishizawa T, Yoshinaka H, Shimazu H: Endorectal ultrasonography for the assessment of wall invasion and lymph node metastasis in rectal cancer. Dis Colon Rectum 1992;35:362–368.
42 Hurlstone DP, Brown S, Cross SS, Shorthouse AJ, Sanders DS: Endoscopic Ultrasound miniprobe staging of colorectal cancer: Can management be modified? Endoscopy 2005;37:710–714.
43 Beynon J, Mortensen NJ, Foy DM, Channer JL, Rigby H, Virjee J: Preoperative assessment of mesorectal lymph node involvement in rectal cancer. Br J Surg 1989;76:276–279.
44 Balthazar EJ, Megibow AJ, Hulnick D, Naidich DP: Carcinoma of the colon: detection and preoperative staging by CT. AJR Am J Roentgenol 1988;150:301–306.
45 Holdsworth PJ, Johnston D, Chalmers AG, Chennells P, Dixon MF, Finan PJ, et al: Endoluminal ultrasound and computed tomography in the staging of rectal cancer. Br J Surg 1988;75:1019–1022.
46 Akasu T, Sugihara K, Moriya Y, Fujita S: Limitations and pitfalls of transrectal ultrasonography for staging of rectal cancer. Dis Colon Rectum 1997;40(suppl):S10–S15.
47 Brown G, Riachards CJ, Bourne MW, et al: Morphologic predictors of lymph node status in rectal cancer with use of high-spatial-resolution MRI with histopathologic comparison. Radiology 2003;227:371–377.
48 Koh DM, Brown G, Temple L, Raja A, Toomey P, Bett N, et al: Rectal cancer: mesorectal lymph nodes at MRI with USPIO versus histopathologic findings – initial observations. Radiology 2004;231:91–99.
49 Taouli B, Vilgrain V, Dumont E, Daire JL, Fan B, Menu Y: Evaluation of liver diffusion anisotropy and characterization of focal hepatic lesions with single-shot echo-planar MRI sequences: prospective study in 66 patients. Radiology 2003;226:71–78.
50 Hein PA, Kremser C, Judmaier W, et al: Diffusion-weighted magnetic resonance imaging for monitoring diffusion changes in rectal carcinoma during combined, preoperative chemoradiation: preliminary results of a prospective study. Eur J Radiol 2003;45:214–222.
51 Shoemaker D, Black R, Giles L, Toouli J: Yearly colonoscopy, liver CT, and chest radiology do not influence 5-year survival of colorectal cancer patients. Gastroenterology 1998;114:7–14.
52 Archer SG, Gray BN: Vascularization of small liver metastases. Br J Surg 1989;76: 545–548.
53 Ridge JA, Bading JR, Gelbard AS, Benua RS, Daly JM: Perfusion of colorectal hepatic metastases. Relative distribution of flow from the hepatic artery and portal vein. Cancer 1987;59:1547–1533.
54 Ackerman NB: Experimental studies on the role of the portal circulation in the hepatic tumour vascularity. Cancer 1986;58:1653–1657.
55 Lin G, Hagerstrand I, Lunderquist A: Portal blood supply of liver metastases. AJR Am J Roentgenol 1984;143:53–55.
56 Lin G, Lunderquist A, Hagerstrand I, Boijsen E: Postmortem examination of the blood supply and vascular pattern of small liver metastases in man. Surgery 1984;96:517–526.
57 Strohmeyer T, Haugeberg G, Lierse W: Angioarchitecture and blood supply of micro- and macrometastases in humans livers. J Hepatol 1987;4:181–189.
58 Sugarbaker PH: Surgical decision making for large bowel cancer metastasis to the liver. Radiology 1990;174:621–626.
59 Hollet MD, Jeffrey RB Jr, Nino-Murcia M, Jorgensen NJ, Harris DP: Dual-phase helical CT of the liver: value of arterial phase scans in the detection of small (<1.5 cm) malignant hepatic neoplasms. AJR Am J Roentgenol 1995;164:879–874.
60 Leen E, Angerson WJ, Wotherspoon H, Moule B, Cooke TG, McArdle CS: Detection of colorectal liver metastases: comparison of laparotomy, CT, US and Doppler Perfusion Index and evaluation of postoperative follow-up results. Radiology 1995;195:113–116.
61 Leen E, Angerson WJ, Cooke TG, McArdle CS: Prognostic Power of Doppler Perfusion Index in colorectal cancer. Correlation with survival. Ann Surg 1996;223:199–203.
62 Wernecke K, Rummeny E, Bongartz G, et al: Detection of hepatic masses in patients with carcinoma: comparative sensitivities of sonography, CT and MRI. AJR Am J Roentgenol 1991;157:731–739.
63 Bleuzen A, Tranquart F: Incidental liver lesions: diagnostic value of cadence contrast pulse sequencing and SonoVue. Eur Radiol 2004;14(suppl 8):P53–P62.
64 Quaia E, Calliada F, Bertolotto M, et al: Characterization of focal liver lesions by contrast-specific US modes and a sulfur hexafluoride-filled microbubble contrast agent: diagnostic performance and confidence. Radiology 2004;232:420–430.
65 Quaia E, Bertolotto M, Forgács B, Rimondini A, Locatelli M, Pozzi Mucelli R: Detection of liver metastases by Pulse Inversion Harmonic Imaging during Levovist late phase: comparison to conventional ultrasound and helical CT in 160 patients. Eur Radiol 2003; 13:475–483.
66 Albrecht T, Blomley MJK, Burns PN, et al: Improved detection of hepatic metastases with pulse-inversion US during the liver-specific phase of SHU 508A: multicenter study. Radiology 2003;227:361–370.
67 Krix M, Plathow C, Essig M, Herfarth K, Debus J, Kauczor HU, Delorme S: Monitoring of liver metastases after stereotactic radiotherapy using low-MI contrast-enhanced ultrasound – initial results. Eur Radiol 2005; 15:677–684.
68 Quaia E, D'Onofrio M, Palumbo A, Rossi S, Bruni S, Cova M: Comparison of contrast-enhanced ultrasonography versus baseline ultrasound and contrast-enhanced computed tomography in metastatic disease of the liver: diagnostic performance and confidence. Eur Radiol 2006;16:1599–1609.
69 Hagspiel KD, Neidel KFW, Eichenberger AC, Weder W, Marincek B: Detection of liver metastases: comparison of superparamagnetic iron-oxide-enhanced MRI at 1.5 T with dynamic CT, intraoperative US, and percutaneous US. Radiology 1995;196:471–478.
70 Ward J, Naik KS, Guthrie JA, Wilson D, Robinson PJ: Hepatic lesion detection: comparison of MRI after the administration of superparamagnetic iron oxide with dual-phase CT by using alternative free response receiver-operating characteristic analysis. Radiology 1999;210:459–466.
71 Bartolozzi C, Donati F, Cioni D, Procacci C, Morana G, Chiesa A, Grazioli L, Cittadini G, Cittadini G, Giovagnoni A, Gandini G, Maass J, Lencioni R: Detection of colorectal liver metastases: a prospective multicenter trial comparing unenhanced MRI, MnDPDP-enhanced MRI, and spiral CT. Eur Radiol 2004;14:14–20.
72 Haider MA, Amitai MM, Rappaport DC, et al: Multi-detector row helical CT in preoperative assessment of small (≤1.5 cm) liver metastases: is thinner collimation better? Radiology 2002;225:137–142.
73 Bipat S, van Leeuwen MS, Comans EF, et al: Colorectal liver metastases: CT, MRI, and PET for diagnosis meta-analysis. Radiology 2005;237:123–131.
74 Bhattacharjya S, Bhattacharjya T, Baber S, Tibballs JM, Watkinson AF, Davidson R: Prospective study of contrast-enhanced computed tomography, computed tomography during arterioportography, and magnetic resonance imaging for staging colorectal liver metastases for liver resection Br J Surg 2004;91:1361–1369.

75 Outwater E, Tomaszewski JE, Daly JM, Kressel HY: Hepatic colorectal metastasis: correlation of MRI and pathologic appearances. Radiology 1991;180:327–332.
76 Imam K, Bluemke DA: MRI in the evaluation of hepatic metastases. Magn Reson Imaging Clin North Am 2000;8:741–756.
77 Kim YK, Ko SW, Hwang SB, Kim CS, Yu HC: Detection and characterization of liver metastases: 16-slice multidetector CT versus superparamagnetic iron oxide-enhanced magnetic resonance imaging. Eur Radiol 2006;16:1337–1345.
78 Leveson SH, Wiggins PA, Nasiru TA, Giles GR, Robinson PJ, Parkin A: Improving the detection of hepatic metastases by the use of dynamic flow scintigraphy. Br J Cancer 1983; 47:719–721.
79 Leveson SH, Wiggins PA, Giles GR, Parkin A, Robinson PJ: Deranged liver blood flow patterns in the detection of liver metastases. Br J Surg 1985;72:128–130.
80 Leen E, Angerson WJ, Wotherspoon H, Moule B, Cooke TG, McArdle CS: Comparison of the Doppler Perfusion Index and intraoperative ultrasonography in diagnosing colorectal liver metastases. Evaluation with postoperative follow-up results. Ann Surg 1994;220:663–667.
81 Yarmenitis SD, Kalogeropoulou CP, Hatjikondi O, et al: An experimental approach of the Doppler Perfusion Index of the liver in detecting occult hepatic metastases: histological findings related to the hemodynamic measurements in Wistar rats. Eur Radiol 2000;10:417–424.
82 Kruskal JB, Thomas P, Kane RA, Goldberg SN: Hepatic perfusion changes in mice livers with developing colorectal cancer metastases. Radiology 2004;231:482–490.

Review Article

Digestive Diseases

Dig Dis 2007;25:33–43
DOI: 10.1159/000099168

Laparoscopic Approach to Colonic Cancer: Critical Appraisal of the Literature

Abe Fingerhut[a] Toufik Ata[a] Elie Chouillard[a] Nicholas Alexakis[b] Nicolas Veyrie[a]

[a]Digestive Surgery Unit, Centre Hospitalier Intercommunal, Poissy, France, and [b]University Department of Surgery, Hippokration Hospital, Athens, Greece

Key Words
Colonic cancer, laparoscopic approach · Laparoscopic colectomy · Laparoscopic colonic resection · Laparoscopic surgery, review of literature

Abstract
Background/Aims: As laparoscopic colectomy finds its place in the surgical armamentarium, the literature concerning the safety, efficacy, and oncological rational for treatment of colonic cancer is also enriched. A review and critical appraisal of the literature on this subject was the aim of this paper. ***Methods:*** A systematic research and a hand search were conducted to gain access to all controlled studies involving laparoscopic colectomy using the Medline, Embase, HealthSTAR, Cumulative Index for Nursing and Allied Health Literature, CancerLit data bases and the Cochrane Central Register of Controlled Trials for the years 1991–2006. ***Results:*** Over 40 controlled randomized trials and ten systematic reviews and/or meta-analyses were found. Several of the completed controlled randomized trials have published either short- or long-term results; only partial and short-term results are available in rectal cancer. The principal conclusions are that the laparoscopic approach affords better short-term outcomes including surgical site morbidity, but with increased operative times and direct costs. Among the proven long-term outcomes, cancer recurrence and survival do not seem to be worse. Whether conversion, a source of increased operative time and costs, is responsible for poorer outcomes or whether specific settings associated with poorer outcomes are among the causes of conversion remains to be shown. However, there are still concerns as regards specific laparoscopic-related complications. ***Conclusion:*** There seems to no real safety problems in performing laparoscopic colectomy for cancer; improvement in operative times, conversion rates, and complications should make laparoscopy the best cost-effective approach to colectomy.

Introduction

Colorectal cancer is the fourth most common cancer in both men and women in the USA [1, 2], and the third and second most common cancer for men and women, respectively, in France [3]. Over 130,000 new cases are diagnosed and approximately 50,000 deaths are attributed to colorectal cancer in the USA each year. In France, over 36,000 new cases, representing 15% of all cancers, are diagnosed every year and slightly more than 16,000 patients die each year of colorectal cancer [3].

In the USA, approximately 160,000 colectomies are performed annually, 107,000 (67%) by the open approach, 28,000 (18%) by the hand-assisted approach, and 25,000 (15%) by the purely laparoscopic approach.

In spite of immense progress in the fields of chemotherapy and immunotherapy, surgical resection remains the mainstay of curative treatment for colorectal cancer.

KARGER
Fax +41 61 306 12 34
E-Mail karger@karger.ch
www.karger.com

0257–2753/07/0251–0033$23.50/0

Accessible online at:
www.karger.com/ddi

A. Fingerhut, MD, FACS, FRCS
Centre Hospitalier Intercommunal
FR–78300 Poissy (France)
Tel. +33 1 3927 5164, Fax +33 1 3927 4402
E-Mail AbeFinger@aol.com

The acceptance of laparoscopic surgery for colonic and rectal cancer, however, has been slow for several reasons: laparoscopic colonic resection (LCR) is technically challenging, involving maneuvers in all four quadrants (retraction of the small bowel and greater omentum, dissection, division of mesenteric blood vessels, and digestive tract anastomosis), new technical skills, the need for extraction of a bulky specimen, along with the use of ever-evolving instrumentation and stapling devices, and finally, fears that LCR could adversely influence outcome. After a shaky start, laparoscopic colorectal surgery is rapidly gaining its credentials, both in benign and now also in malignant disease. The goal of this paper was to cull and review the current literature concerning the laparoscopic approach to colonic cancer, and to critically appraise the available evidence.

Material and Methods

To gain access to all publications, and especially the controlled randomized trials, systematic reviews, and meta-analyses involving laparoscopic (vs. open) colectomy and rectal resections, we performed a systematic research of the electronic literature using the Medline, Embase, HealthSTAR, Cumulative Index for Nursing and Allied Health Literature, CancerLit data bases and the Cochrane Central Register of Controlled Trials for the years 1991–2006. The search strategy was that described by Dickersin and colleagues [4, 5] with the appropriate specific search terms for 'colectomy', 'colonic resection', 'colon', 'intestine-large', 'colonic neoplasm', 'rectum', 'rectal resection', 'proctectomy', 'laparosc*', and 'controlled trials'.

Additionally, the following journals were hand searched: *American Journal of Surgery, Archives of Surgery, Annals of Surgery, British Journal of Surgery, Disease of Colon and Rectum, International Journal of Colorectal Disease, Journal of American College of Surgeons* (formerly *Surgery, Gynecology and Obstetrics*), *Journal of Gastrointestinal Surgery, Lancet, Langenbeck's Archives of Surgery, Surgical Endoscopy, Surgical Laparoscopic Endoscopy, Surgery*, and the *World Journal of Surgery*.

Results

Over 40 controlled randomized trials were found. Of note, at least eight publications contained duplicated information [6–13] and were not analyzed further. Several other publications were deemed unfit for analysis because of absence of clinical data [14], faulty randomization [15] and three other trials because they involved different anastomotic techniques during laparoscopic sigmoidectomy [16] or compared hand-assisted laparoscopy to laparoscopy [17] and differences between gasless laparoscopy and pneumoperitoneum during laparoscopic colectomy [18].

Ten systematic reviews and/or meta-analyses were found [19–28].

Among the controlled randomized trials underway in the world, several have been published, either as long-term [29–33] or short-term results [34–37]. Several other publications have dealt with partial results, or specific issues of these same or other individual studies [38–46].

As concerns rectal cancer, there are only partial and short-term results available in two trials [34, 39], and we did not analyze the results further.

The major conclusion of these studies is that feasibility of laparoscopic colectomy has been shown to be safe, with advantageous immediate surgical site complications (compared to open colectomy), reasonable morbidity and mortality, as well as long-term carcinological outcomes. The probability of less incisional hernia in the long term, as well as the ease of repair of trocar incisional hernia, compared with the difficult and recurrence-prone repair of incisional hernia after open colectomy may prove to be the major advantage of laparoscopic colectomy. Conversions rate range between 11 and 29% in the randomized controlled trials. Conversion leads to increased operative times and costs. Whether conversion is responsible for poorer outcomes or whether specific settings associated with poorer outcomes are among the causes of conversion remains to be shown. However, there are still concerns as regards increased costs, including longer operative times, and specific laparoscopic-related complications.

Discussion

The safety and technical feasibility of LCR has slowly been confirmed [47–49]. Several non-randomized [50–61] as well as randomized studies [30–36] have underscored that the minimal invasive approach to colectomy decreased postoperative pain with reduction in narcotic usage, and lead to earlier ambulation, faster return to bowel function and oral intake, as well as earlier hospital discharge.

Most of the above-mentioned benefits, however, although reproducible, are modest. Moreover, these classical endpoints were not used in most studies to calculate the power of their trials, and therefore the use of these endpoints to demonstrate the superiority of one technique over the other is highly debatable.

Comparative studies whose design allows patients to have different pain scores just because they are in one or another arm are ethically criticizable: all efforts today should be concentrated on reducing postoperative pain for all patients. The differences could then be the quantity of analgesics necessary so that pain scores would be minimal but equal. When, however, the results of the studies that looked at the difference in the quantity of analgesics necessary are analyzed, the differences were minimal without much clinical relevance: no statistically significant difference in the EORTC pain scores [34], difference of 1 day (median) in duration of parenteral narcotic or oral analgesic use [33], difference of 2.4 injections of morphine (mean) less on day 1 [32], difference of 3–14 of 1,082 patients requiring analgesic use [36]. Patients should be blinded to the approach (never mentioned in any of the controlled randomized trials).

Faster return to bowel function and oral intake has long been highlighted as an advantage of the laparoscopic approach over the open technique. Recent studies seem to indicate, however, that the difference in postoperative recovery may be less significant when perioperative care is optimized [38, 43, 46, 62]. Clearly, fast-track programs have shown that early return of bowel function and oral intake can be achieved even with open colectomy [38, 62, 63]. The same is true for the use of thoracic epidural anesthesia-analgesia [43]. Two recent randomized trials have provided contradictory results. Basse et al. [38], in a study of 60 patients, did not find any significant difference in postoperative recovery parameters. On the other hand, a more recent study by King et al. [42] showed that there was a shorter recovery period and hospital stay when fast-track or enhanced recovery care was instigated in LCR. In a recent systematic review [64], the combined results of six papers (three randomized controlled and three controlled clinical trials), including 512 patients found that both the primary hospital stay and morbidity (relative risk 0.54, 95% CI 0.42–0.69) were significantly lower for such programs. Higher readmission rates, on the other hand, a potential trade-off for shorter hospital stay, were not significantly different (relative risk 1.17, 95% CI 0.73–1.86). Mortality was not found to be increased. Last, the subjectivity that is used to determine hospital discharge is a confounding factor that cannot be ignored any longer. This criterion is of limited value unless the person who decides the hospital discharge (and probably the patient as well) was blinded to the type of approach that was allocated. This has not been reported as such in the case of any of the randomized trials.

Laparoscopy and Cancer

Surgical resection remains the gold standard to cure colon cancer. LCR must be able to achieve the same oncological resection attained by open resection. The problems today are how to reduce the conversion rate, maintaining a high-quality oncological resection, while containing costs.

Conversion

The conversion rate for laparoscopic surgery has been reported to range from 4.2% [65] to 77% [66, 67]. The conversion rate in the controlled randomized trials ranges between 4.2 and 29% [31–34, 36, 39].

Several authors have found that the conversion rate decreased with experience [47, 68]. In a historical control study, Schwandner et al. [69] reported conversion rates of 9.3% for the first 150 procedures and 5.3% for the second 150 operations. In the retrospective multicenter German survey of 1,658 patients, Marusch et al. [68] found that surgeons with experience involving more man 100 laparoscopic colonic operations were more likely to embark on more difficult cases with a conversion rate of 4.3%, as compared with 6.9% for surgeons with experience involving fewer than 100 procedures. Surgeon seniority or experience, represented by the number of operations performed, was established as an independent risk factor for conversion by Tekkis et al. [70]: junior surgeons were shown to be 1.5 times more likely to convert to an open procedure, after adjustment for other confounding variables. On the other hand, according to the data analyzed by Gervaz et al. [66], surgeon experience seems to have little influence on the overall rate of conversion, at least in the studies included in their meta-analysis.

The potentially adverse effects of conversion have been highlighted ever since the report of Slim et al. [71]. These include worse morbidity and mortality [71, 72], worse outcome [34], increased operative time, prolonged hospital stay [72], poorer survival [28, 36, 73], increased need for transfusion [34], and increased costs [40]. While it is certainly possible that these poor outcomes were the consequence of conversion, it might also be that the reasons for conversion could possibly have a part in determining these adverse outcomes, for instance, a large tumor, adhering to the abdominal wall, considered as a poor prognostic factor, could be the cause for conversion. Two groups have looked at independent risk factors for conversion [70, 74]. Both found that increased BMI and surgeon experience were independent risk factors. The other independent risk factors found included malignancy [74] and type of resection (low rectal, left colorectal, right colonic vs. small/other bowel procedures and presence of intraoperative abscess [70]. Of note, abscess and fistula as related to perforation carry a particularly worse influence on prognosis [75].

The recommendations of Belizon et al. [72] warrant reflection: prompt conversion to open (<30 min into operation) significantly reduced postoperative morbidity which leads some to distinguish between early (<30 min) and late (>30 min) conversions [72]. The former are due to difficulties in access, intraoperative discovery of contraindication to LCR (see later), or early complications. The latter are essentially due to (late) intraoperative complications, impossibility to perform the anastomosis or extract the specimen.

Although some of the conversion rates may be considered by some as high, the conversion rates listed in such controlled trials have to be considered as representative of results of the average surgeon performing laparoscopic surgery in our era. Moreover, as underscored by Gervaz et al. [66], when a precise definition is used to define what the authors mean by conversion, the rate is always and statistically significantly higher than when the opposite is true. However, it is difficult to assess the conversion rate as such, and to compare the rate between studies, because of lack of a standard definition. As well, it is difficult if not impossible to take into consideration the variability of surgical skill, experience, and subjectivity which is so important in determining when the surgeon decides to 'convert'.

As concerns the definition, Tekkis et al. [70] proposed talking about conversion when there was a need for a midline laparotomy >10 cm, for either completion of the operative procedure or extraction of the specimen. Casillas et al. [76], once masses >10 cm had been eliminated, defined conversion as any incision >10 cm, or operating through the incision if <10 cm. Others consider conversion to mean any incision exceeding 7 cm [39]. Still others [47, 50] have used a much vaguer definition: 'deviation from the operative plan requiring a major abdominal incision to complete the procedure', or 'an unplanned laparotomy (median laparotomy and Pfannenstiel incision) or an incision made longer or earlier than planned (6 cm is implied) [69].

One paper [49] went to greater details to avoid the use of an incision length in the definition of conversion and to subdue the subjectivity in the decision to 'convert': these authors defined conversion as any operation during which mobilization of the colon and its mesentery or performance of the anastomosis requires additional length of incision (including widening the incision necessary to extract the specimen), or, without extension of the incision, when 'additional mobilization or unsuspected steps' are necessary to complete the operation.

Oncological Quality of Laparoscopic Resections

By convention, the oncological adequacy of resection for colon cancer is defined by the parameters of *length of bowel resected to yield tumor-free margins* and the *number of lymph nodes* harvested in the specimen. Curative resection is often expressed as a R0 resection (no macroscopically visible tumor left behind) [77]. Several randomized studies [31–33, 44] have shown that laparoscopy can achieve the same curative resection as open surgery. In the meta-analysis by Korolija et al. [23], which looked at 35 studies with data on lymph node count and distal margin clearance (total of 3,935 patients) published between 1990 and 1999, including 16 comparative studies, 6 open series, and 13 laparoscopic series, the average distal margin clearance was 4.6 cm with the laparoscopic approach and 5.3 cm with the open approach. This difference was statistically significant in favor of the open approach. Further, there were more lymph nodes extracted laparoscopically (0.3–2.14 more). This difference was statistically significant only for the fixed-effects single-outcome model; as these studies were heterogeneous in quality, this is somewhat methodologically debatable. Schwenk et al. [26], in their meta-analysis, considered only the results of seven randomly controlled trials (688 participants) and found that there were no significant differences between the two groups either as concerned the length of resected specimen (2 trials, 134 cancer patients) (weighted mean difference (WMD): 0.71 [95% CI –2.05 to 3.48; p = 0.61] or the number of lymph nodes: RR = 0.12 [95% CI –1.17 to 1.41; p = 0.86]), thus confirming the findings of Korolija et al. [23], but with sounder methodology.

In addition to the resection of the primary cancer, surgical exploration should provide valuable additional information as to the stage of the cancer. Clinically and radiologically unrecognized peritoneal metastases can be as easily identified and biopsied during laparoscopic surgery as in open resection [24]. On the other hand, accurate detection of liver involvement through preoperative imaging studies, such as computed tomography (CT), CT arterial portography, and magnetic resonance imaging with and without injection of contrast material, while improving at a rapid rate, still lack sensitivity for small lesions in the liver [78–80]. Intraoperative laparoscopic ultrasound has been touted to fill the void left by the inability to palpate the liver at laparoscopy [81, 82]. Of note, however, unsuspected tumor invasion or inadequate preoperative evaluation was the reason for conversion in 25 of 435 (28% of conversions) [33], 20 of 167 (43% of conversions) [32], 52 of 536 (57% of conversions) [36] and 40 of 246 (66% of conversions) [34] patients in the controlled studies, respectively. This underscores the need for better workup before embarking on laparoscopic resection for all-comers.

Surgical Site or Port-Site Recurrences

The ominous report by Berends et al. [83], who reported a 21% incidence of port-site recurrences and raised the possibility that the pneumoperitoneum somehow altered the pattern of spread and local wound biology, created great concern in the laparoscopic surgical community [84]. Several other studies of different size and design have also dealt with wound recurrence after laparoscopic resections [6, 9, 31, 51, 54, 56, 58, 61, 85–89]. More recent data from large series (single institutions with over 100 patients and multi-institution series with over 400 patients), however, showed that the wound recurrence rate was in reality between 0 and 2.4%, somewhat comparable to what had been reported in open colectomy, ranging from 0.9 to 3.3% [35, 78, 87, 90–92]. At least five prospective randomized trials have shown that the incidence of wound recurrence was not a major issue [27, 31, 33, 36, 44].

Survival

As we are dealing with cancer, survival should be the major endpoint. Three-year survival data are now available for at least four controlled randomized trials [31–34]. In this chapter we will review the data of three of these trials [31–33], criticizing their strong points and weaknesses.

Among the trials presently available for analysis, the Barcelona trial [31] was designed as an 'equivalency' trial; the COST trial [33] was a 'non-inferiority' trial, whereas the Hong Kong [32], COLOR [36], and the CLASICC [34] studies were designed as 'superiority' trials.

Except for the Lacy study, the RCT have shown that laparoscopic colectomy is at least equivalent to open colectomy as concerns oncological surgery. Short-term advantages include fewer surgical site complications, and were touted to require fewer analgesics with better short-term convalescence. However, all laparoscopic procedures took longer to perform.

In fact, all these trials have several important shortcomings that warrant mention. Three RCT [31, 32, 39] were monocenter studies, and as such, results are perhaps not applicable to other surgical populations, or other surgical teams. The COST, COLOR and CLASICC trials were multicenter studies, and wide applicability is therefore better fitted.

The Lacy study, the only one to show any statistically significant difference in cancer-related survival, was severely criticized for several methodological flaws [93–95], which along with some personal remarks, are summarized hereafter. Let it be said that the response by Lacy [96] was hardly convincing. The main criticisms include: (1) Partial results of the same patient population were published in other publications [9] (91 patients included from November 1993 through January 1996) before the final results were published in *Lancet* in 2002 perhaps influencing the way patients, and assessors, envisioned the follow-up period. (2) Inconsistencies between the previous, partially published results and the final paper in 2002 including: (a) difference in the number of exclusions because of distant metastases (20 [9] vs. 11 [31]); (b) differences in the number or overlap of recruitment periods [7, 97], and (c) differences in the indications for patients receiving chemotherapy: Dukes' stage B2 and C only [9] vs. routine chemotherapy for stages II and III [31]. (3) Of 442 eligible patients, only 219 were randomized. While the reasons for not including these patients in the study are given, no information as to their outcome was provided. (4) Postoperative chemotherapy was administered to 68 (61%) in the laparoscopic group and to 59 (55%) in the conventional group (difference statistically nonsignificant but lopsided in the same direction as the favorable outcome) and not included in the multivariate analysis, to determine whether it was an independent variable or not. On the other hand, adjuvant chemotherapy was given to 68 of 79 stage II or III patients in the laparoscopy group, but only to 59 of 84 stage II and III patients in the conventional group ($p = 0.023$, two-sided Fisher's exact test) which might have influenced the outcome. (5) Further oncological concerns include: (a) absence of reported complete (R0) tumor resection rate (especially since there were twice as many patients with T4 tumors in the conventional group), (b) absence of outcome in patients with liver metastases (excluded after randomization) or with locally incomplete tumor resection. (6) Other methodological concerns include: (a) failure to mention the upper and lower limits of the two-sided interval characteristic of the equivalence study, (b) subgroup analysis to state that laparoscopic treatment was better than open, and (c) (if we admit that cancer-free survival is the complement of 100% cancer-related death) the actual difference in cancer-free survival was

(100–9 =) 91% – (100–21 =) 79% = 12%, well under the 15% interval the authors set up to determine that there was a difference, (d) analysis did not adhere to the intention-to-treat principle. (7) Finally, no autopsies seemed to have been performed to ensure that the patients deceased were for reasons unrelated to carcinoma.

The Clinical Outcomes of Surgical Therapy Study Group, or COST study [33], a multicenter, non-inferiority trial, found that there was no statistically significant difference at 3 years in the rates of recurrence (16% for LCR vs. 18% OC; two-sided $p = 0.32$; hazard ratio for recurrence, 0.86; 95% CI 0.63–1.17), the overall survival rate (86 vs. 85%, respectively; $p = 0.51$), or the time to recurrence or overall survival irrespective of the stage of cancer.

Among the criticisms reported [98], we note: (1) absence of definition of the non-inferiority boundary ($-\Delta$ to 0); (2) the statistical methods used correspond to failed superiority trial, and (3) if one considers non-inferiority to be when the upper limit of the one-sided 95% CI for hazard ratio is less than the non-inferiority boundary, the conclusion could be that there was as much as a 16% increase in risk of death and a 11% increase in risk of recurrence in the laparoscopic group. Moreover, it is not clear how many patients had their anastomosis performed laparoscopically.

The monocenter Leung study [32] involved only left-sided cancer. In this superiority trial, the authors found no significant differences in the probabilities of survival at 5 years (76.1% (standard error of the mean: 3.7%) and 72.9% (4.0%), respectively), of being disease-free at 5 years (75.3% (3.7%) and 78.3% (3.7%), respectively). The 95% CI for the difference in 5-year survival was –7.5 to 13.9%, compatible outcome for laparoscopic resection ranging from 7.5% worse survival to 13.9% better survival than open resection. The difference sought was 15%, only just outside the confidence interval. Once again, the number of patients at risk at 5 years was 104 or 104/403 = 26%.

Of note, the number of patients available for 5-year follow-up in these three trials was 25.7%. Both of these trials [31, 33], as well as the COLOR and CLASICC studies for which only short-term results are available, included a high proportion of right colectomies (47% for the Lacy trial, 54% for the COST trial, 47% for the COLOR, and 46% for the 313 colonic resections in the CLASICC trial). Right colectomy differs greatly from left colectomy in its performance, oncological tactics, immediate outcome, and difficulties [99–101].

The Braga study [29] did not provide the necessary calculations as to the number of patients necessary. There were no statistically significant differences in overall or disease-free survival.

All in all, while there certainly is a tendency to show that survival is at least not worse with LCR, the methodological flaws in these studies are such that they do not allow to reach these conclusions yet, but only to infer that these outcomes are true. Longer and more complete follow-up results are eagerly awaited for these trials.

Costs, Quality of Life following Hospital Discharge, and Long-Term Surgical-Site Outcomes

Costs

Of the studies available in the literature, most were cost-minimization studies. While some have found that costs were increased by laparoscopic colectomy relative to open colectomy (difference in AUD 1,183 ($p = 0.001$) [102], difference in USD 2,000 ($p = 0.02$) [103]), three of the studies, which looked at direct costs, gave quite different results. One study [104] found an advantage for laparoscopic surgery of USD 3,655 – 3,299 = 356 ($p = 0.0034$), another [42] found no difference, while a third, the Hong Kong study [32], found that laparoscopic surgery was USD 2,149 more expensive ($p < 0.001$).

Two cost minimization studies looked at subsets of the COLOR (n = 210) [41] and CLASICC (n = 682) [40]. Both confirmed that operative and overall costs were higher in LRC. Other hospital (non-OR) costs were lower in LCR. Other findings included: higher average cost to individuals for reoperations in LCR, cost of first admission, and total cost to the healthcare system. In another cost minimization study, King et al. [42] compared short-term outcomes of 62 patients, demographically similar, randomized on a 2:1 basis to receive laparoscopic (n = 43) or open (n = 19) resection of colorectal cancer within an enhanced recovery program. The length of hospital stay ($p = 0.018$), the combined hospital, convalescent, and readmission stay ($p = 0.012$) were shorter for LCR.

Two cost-benefit analyses, one randomized [105] and the other retrospective [106], concluded the LCR took longer to perform, hospital stay was shorter. The randomized study showed that overall morbidity rate was better after LCR 18.2 versus 34.7% ($p < 0.0005$) and that the better postoperative short-term outcome in patients receiving LCR played a key role to nearly balance the operative room charges due to laparoscopy [105]. The second [106] showed that total hospital costs were significantly lower for LCR compared with open colectomy and that LCR was cost-effective resulting in significant savings to the healthcare system.

These five papers are important because they underline that LCR should provide great benefits both to the patient and to the healthcare systems, as long as the complication rate stays low, and probably, also, if an enhanced recovery program is used. However, as concerns the shorter hospital stay taken individually, no conclusions can be made, as it is well known that without blinding, hospital discharge should not be used as a surrogate for recovery. This was the main criticism for all the abovementioned studies.

Quality of Life

In the COST trial [37], one of the earliest to look at this aspect, data for 449 consecutive patients with clinically resectable colon cancer showed better global rating scale scores for 2 weeks postsurgery in LCR vs. OC ($p = 0.009$). While in the hospital, patients assigned to LCR (vs. OC) required fewer days of both parenteral analgesics ($p < 0.001$) and oral analgesics ($p = 0.03$). The short-term quality of life (QOL) benefit was statistically and very moderately clinically significant in LCR at 2 weeks only. Later, these benefits disappeared.

Janson [107] assessed the QOL in patients from the COLOR trial using a cancer-specific questionnaire. The laparoscopic patients fared better on the social functioning component of the EORTC QLQ-30 score at 2 and 4 weeks and on the role function component at 2 weeks.

Braga et al. [29] also looked at QOL as related to long-term complications and survival rate ($n = 391$). Overall QOL was significantly better in the LCR during the first 12 months after surgery, associated with a lower incidence of long-term complications, whereas at 24 months LCR patients reported a significant advantage only in social functioning.

In the CLASICC multicenter clinical trial [34], EORTC QLQ-C30 scores for global QOL and functional scales showed that there was no significant difference at 2 weeks and 3 months.

Possible reasons for this disparity in results include the accrual mode, which was selective in the Weeks study [37], perhaps introducing a selection bias, as well as the fact that in the COST study, the number of inclusions per center was low compared with the COLOR study.

Additional advantages of the laparoscopic route for colectomy include effective palliative resection for patients with locally advanced, or stage 4 cancer [30, 108], laparoscopic stoma confection in these same patients with locally advanced or recurrent cancer, allowing commencement of chemoradiation treatment as rapidly as possible [109]. The avoidance of a major laparotomy in this setting is clearly desirable.

Most likely, one of the until now little publicized advantages of laparoscopic surgery should logically be less long-term surgical site morbidity, that is less postoperative incisional hernia. Although there is no grade 1 evidence to substantiate this claim, let it be said that most authors admit a 1–19% incisional hernia rate for all surgical site wounds [110, 111], but some have reported as high as a 20% rate for colonic interventions [45], depending on the quality and length of follow-up. The published rates of incision hernia after laparoscopic surgery range between 0.65 and 2.80% overall [112, 113] and between 0.6 [114] and 4.7% [29] for colorectal disease. Of note, one study [45] looked at 83 patients in their institution participating in a large multicenter randomized trial (37 LCR and 46 OCR). Seven patients in the LCR group had been converted to OCR. Surgical site infections occurred in 13.5% of patients after LCR (2.7% trocar, 10.8% extraction sites) and in 10.9% of patients after OCR. During a mean follow-up of 30.1 ± 17.8 months, incisional hernias developed in 24.3% of patients after LCR and in 17.4% after OCR. In the LCR group, extraction sites accounted for 85.7% of all wound complications. The authors concluded that the extraction site for LCR was associated with a high incidence of complications, comparable to open colectomy, and stressed that strategies to alter operative technique should be considered to reduce the incidence of these complications.

Future Endeavors

Long-term results are needed for all of the patients entered into the randomized trials. Efforts have been made to lump together the outcomes of the Lacy, COST, CLASICC, and COLOR trials, as concerns the short-term, and soon, hopefully the long-term survival outcomes. Trials are needed to indicate the best way to decrease the operating time and other direct costs that plague laparoscopic colectomy for the moment. For these reasons, four further controlled randomized studies [115–118] warrant closer analysis.

Marcello et al. [115] compared laparoscopic vascular staplers and disposable clip appliers with the LigaSure Atlas during elective right, left, and total colectomy (152 vessels ligated vs. 169 vessels sealed with the LigaSure).

Table 1. Outcomes according to four controlled randomized studies [115–118]

	Targarona et al. [118]	Morino et al. [116]	Marcello et al. [115]	Takada et al. [117]
Comparison	ES: dissection with ES, vessels clipped vs. CBBE completed by 10-mm LIG vs. 5-mm UC for bowel dissection, vascular pedicle dissection, and mesocolon transaction Mesenteric vessel pedicle controlled with endostapler	UC vs. standard ES	S/C vs. LIG	CBBE vs. US
Number of patients (pts); vessels (v)	38 pts	171 pts	48 pts 152 v vs. 52 pts 169 v	30 pts
Failure/rebleeding			14 (9.2%) of 152 vs. 5 (3%) of 169	0.3 vs. 1.2 (TC); 0.3 vs. 2.0 (Sig)
Blood loss	Less with conventional ES vs. UC or CBBE	UC 140.8 ml vs. ES 182.6 ml (p = 0.032	50 ml (20–50) vs. 100 ml (25–800) (p = 0.054)	
Costs	NS		USD 317 ± 0 vs. USD 400 ± 112 (p < 0.001)	
Operative time	Longer with conventional ES vs. UC or CBBE	UC 93 min vs. ES 102.6 min (p = 0.46)		7.9 vs. 18.4 min, 15.0 vs. 27.6 min

ES = Electrosurgery; UC = ultracision (harmonic scapel); S/C = vascular staplers and disposable clip appliers; LIG = LigaSure Atlas; CBBE = computed-based bipolar energy; TC = transverse colectomy; Sig = sigmoidectomy.

Morino et al. [116] assessed the safety and efficacy of the ultrasonic dissection (UC) compared with standard electrosurgery (ES) in 171 patients undergoing laparoscopic colorectal surgery. Takada et al. [117] compared the effectiveness of three different energy sources on the laparoscopic performance of a left colectomy in 38 non-selected patients requiring an elective segmental left-sided colon resection: ES plus clips; bipolar ES completed by 10-mm LigaSure; 5-mm ultrasonic shears (Harmonic Scalpel). Targarona et al. [118] conducted a comparative study in 30 patients with colon cancer who underwent laparoscopic colectomy using either the electrothermal bipolar vessel sealer (EBVS) or the ultrasonic coagulating shears (UCS).

Outcomes are provided in table 1. Operative time was shorter when the ultrasonic device (US) or EBVS were used vs. electrocoagulation and vessel clips [117], and when EBVS was compared to the UCS (US) [118]. Blood loss was less when US or EBVS were used vs. electrocoagulation and vessel clips [117], when EBVS was used vs. vascular staplers and clips [115] and when US was used vs. standard ES [116], and less rebleeding when EBVS was compared with vascular staplers and clips [115] or US [118].

In conclusion, energy-driven devices, although they may increase direct costs, are valuable tools to help keep the morbidity to a minimum.

Conclusions

There is now sufficient evidence to show that laparoscopic colectomy is feasible and safe, when performed without excessive complication rates and according to sound oncological principles. The immediate benefits seem to be real, but marginal. Long-term surgical site benefits are probable but remain to be proven. The specter of inordinate surgical site recurrence is no longer a major concern for laparoscopic surgery. The oncological outcome following laparoscopic resections seems at least equivalent to that after open colectomy. All must be done to reduce costs, operative times and conversion rates, and immediate morbidity so that the long-term advantages may surface.

References

1 Ries L, Wingo P, Rosenberg H, Miller D, Howe H, Weir H, Vernon S, Edwards B: The annual report to the nation on the status of cancer, 1973–1997, with a special section on colorectal cancer. Cancer 2000;88:2398–2424.
2 Electronic citation: www.cancer.gov (2006).
3 Selke B, Durand I, Marissal J, Chevalier D, Lebrun T: Cost of colorectal cancer in France in 1999 (in French). Gastroenterol Clin Biol 2003;27:22–27.
4 Dickersin K, Scherer R, Lefebvre C: Identifying relevant studies for systematic reviews. BMJ 1994;309:1286–1291.
5 Tumber M, Dickersin K: Publication of clinical trials: accountability and accessibility. J Int Med 2004;256:271–283.
6 Bohm B, Schwenk W, Muller J: Long-term results after laparoscopic resection of colorectal carcinoma (in German). Chirurg 1999;70:453–455.
7 Delgado S, Lacy A, Filella X, Castells A, Garcia-Valdecasas J, Pique J, Momblan D, Visa J: Acute phase response in laparoscopic and conventional colectomy in colon cancer: a randomised study. Dis Colon Rectum 2001; 44:638–646.
8 Lacy A, Garcia-Valdecasas J, Pique J, Delgado S, Campo E, Bondas J, Taura P, Graude L, Fuster J, Pacheco J, Visa J: Short-term outcome analysis of a randomised study comparing laparoscopic vs. open colectomy for colon cancer. Surg Endosc 1995;9:1101–1105.
9 Lacy A, Delgado S, Garcia-Valdecasas J, Castells A, Pique J, Grande L, Fuster J, Targarona E, Pera M, Visa J: Port site metastases and recurrence after laparoscopic colectomy: a randomized trial. Surg Endosc 1998;12: 1039–1042.
10 Ordemann J, Jacobi C, Schwenck W, Stosslein R, Muller J: Cellular and humoral inflammatory response after laparoscopic and conventional colonic resections. Surg Endosc 2001;15:600–608.
11 Schwenk W, Bohm B, Haase O, Junghans T, Muller J: Laparoscopic versus conventional colorectal resection: a prospective randomised study of postoperative ileus and early postoperative feeding. Langenbecks Arch Surg 1998;383:49–55.
12 Schwenk W, Bohm B, Muller J: Postoperative pain and fatigue after laparoscopic or conventional colorectal resections. A prospective randomized trial. Surg Endosc 1998;12: 1131–1136.
13 Schwenk W, Bohm B, Witt C, Junghans T, Grundel K, Muller J: Pulmonary function following laparoscopic or conventional colorectal resection: a randomized controlled evaluation. Arch Surg 1999;134:6–12.
14 Kim S, Milsom J, Gramlich T, Toddy S, Shore G, Okuda J, Fazio V: Does laparoscopic vs. conventional surgery increase exfoliated cancer cells in the peritoneal cavity during resection of colorectal cancer? Dis Colon Rectum 1998;41:971–978.
15 Hotokezaka M, Dix J, Mentis E, Minasi J, Schirmer B: Gastrointestinal recovery following laparoscopic vs. open colon surgery. Surg Endosc 1996;10:485–489.
16 Bergamaschi R, Tuech J, Cervi C, Arnaud J: Re-establish peumoperitoneum in laparoscopic-assisted sigmoid resection? Dis Colon Rectum 2000;43:771–774.
17 Targarona E, Gracia E, Garriga J, Martinez-Bru C, Cortes M, Boluda R, Lerma L, Trias M: Prospective randomized trial comparing conventional laparoscopic colectomy with hand-assisted laparoscopic colectomy: applicability, immediate clinical outcome, inflammatory response, and cost. Surg Endosc 2002;16:234–239.
18 Schulze S, Lyng K, Bugge K, Perner A, Bendtsen A, Thorup J, Nielsen H, Rasmussen V, Rosenberg J: Cardiovascular and respiratory changes and convalescence in laparoscopic colonic surgery: comparison between carbon dioxide pneumoperitoneum and gasless laparoscopy. Arch Surg 1999;134:1112–1118.
19 Abraham N, Young J, Solomon M: Meta-analysis of short-term outcomes after laparoscopic resection for colorectal cancer. Br J Surg 2004;91:1111–1124.
20 Chapman A, Levitt M, Hewett P, Woods R, Sheiner H, Maddern G: Laparoscopic-assisted resection of colorectal malignancies: a systematic review. Ann Surg 2001;234:590–606.
21 Davies M, Larson D: Laparoscopic surgery for colorectal cancer: the state of the art. Surg Oncol 2004;13:111–118.
22 Kieran J, Curet M: Laparoscopic colon resection for colon cancer. J Surg Res 2004;117: 79–91.
23 Korolija D, Tadic S, Simic D: Extent of oncological resection in laparoscopic vs. open colorectal surgery: meta-analysis. Langenbecks Arch Surg 2003;387:366–371.
24 Luck A, Hensman C, Hewett P: Laparoscopic colectomy for cancer: a review. Aust NZ J Surg 1998;68:318–327.
25 Reza M, Blasco J, Andradas E, Cantero R, Mayol J: Systematic review of laparoscopic versus open surgery for colorectal cancer. Br J Surg 2006;93:921–928.
26 Schwenk W, Haase O, Neudecker J, Muller J: Short-term benefits for laparoscopic colorectal resection. Cochrane Database Syst Rev 2005;3:CD003145.
27 Tjandra J, Chan M: Systematic review on the short-term outcome of laparoscopic resection for colon and rectosigmoid cancer. Colorectal Dis 2006;8:375–388.
28 Yong L, Deane M, Monson J, Darzi A: Systematic review of laparoscopic surgery for colorectal malignancy. Surg Endosc 2001;15: 1431–1439.
29 Braga M, Frasson M, Vignali A, Zuliani W, Civelli V, Di Carlo V: Laparoscopic vs. open colectomy in cancer patients: long-term complications, quality of life, and survival. Dis Colon Rectum 2005;48:2217–2223.
30 Hasegawa H, Kabeshima Y, Watanabe M, Yamamoto S, Kitajima M: Randomized controlled trial of laparoscopic versus open colectomy for advanced colorectal cancer. Surg Endosc 2003;17:636–640.
31 Lacy A, Garcia-Valdecasas J, Delgado S, Castells A, Taura P, Pique J, Visa J: Laparoscopic-assisted colectomy vs. open colectomy for treatment of non-metastatic colon cancer: a randomized trial. Lancet 2002;359:2224–2229.
32 Leung K, Kwok S, Lam S, Lee J, Yiu R, Ng S, Lai P, Lau W: Laparoscopic resection of rectosigmoid carcinoma: prospective randomised trial. Lancet 2004;363:1187–1192.
33 The Clinical Outcomes of Surgical Therapy Study Group: A comparison of laparoscopically-assisted and open colectomy for colon cancer. N Eng J Med 2004;350:2050–2059.
34 Guillou P, Quirke P, Thorpe H, Walker J, Jayne D, Smith A, Heath R, Brown J: Short-term endpoints of conventional versus laparoscopic-assisted surgery in patients with colorectal cancer (MRC CLASICC trial): multicentre, randomised controlled trial. Lancet 2005;365:1718–1726.
35 Milsom J, Bohm B, Hammerhofer K, Fazio V, Steiger E, Elson P: A prospective, randomised trial comparing laparoscopic versus conventional techniques in colorectal cancer surgery: a preliminary report. J Am Coll Surg 1998;187:46–55.
36 Veldkamp R, Kuhry E, Hop W, Jeekel J, Kazemier G, Bonjer H, Haglind E, Pahlman L, Cuesta M, Msika S, Morino M, Lacy A: Laparoscopic surgery versus open surgery for colon cancer: short-term outcomes of a randomised trial. Lancet Oncol 2005;6:477–484.
37 Weeks J, Nelson H, Gelber S, Sargent D, Schroeder G: Short-term quality-of-life outcomes following laparoscopic-assisted colectomy vs. open colectomy for colon cancer: a randomised trial. JAMA 2002;287:321–328.
38 Basse L, Jakobsen D, Bardram L, Billesbolle P, Lund C, Mogensen T, Rosenberg J, Kehlet H: Functional recovery after open versus laparoscopic colonic resection: a randomized, blinded study. Ann Surg 2005;241:416–423.
39 Braga M, Vignali A, Gianotti L, Zuliani W, Radaelli G, Gruarin P, Dellabona P, Di Carlo V: Laparoscopic versus open colorectal surgery: a randomized trial on short-term outcome. Ann Surg 2002;236:759–766.

40 Franks P, Bosanquet N, Thorpe H, Brown J, Copeland J, Smith A, Quirke P, Guillou P: Short-term costs of conventional vs. laparoscopic-assisted surgery in patients with colorectal cancer (MRC CLASICC trial). Br J Cancer 2006;95:6–12.
41 Janson M, Bjorholt I, Carlsson P, Haglind E, Henriksson M, Lindholm E, Anderberg B: Randomized clinical trial of the costs of open and laparoscopic surgery for colonic cancer. Br J Surg 2004;91:409–417.
42 King P, Blazeby J, Ewings P, Franks P, Longman R, Kendrick A, Kipling R, Kennedy R: Randomized clinical trial comparing laparoscopic and open surgery for colorectal cancer within an enhanced recovery program. Br J Surg 2006;93:300–308.
43 Senagore A, Delaney C, Mekhail N, Dugan A, Fazio V: Randomized clinical trial comparing epidural anaesthesia and patient-controlled analgesia after laparoscopic segmental colectomy. Br J Surg 2006;90: 1195–1199.
44 Stage J, Schulze S, Moller P, Overgaard H, Andersen M, Rebsdorfpedersen V, Nielsen H: Prospective randomised study of laparoscopic vs. open colonic resection for adenocarcinoma. Br J Surg 1997;84:391–396.
45 Winslow E, Fleshman J, Birnbaum E, Brunt L: Wound complications of laparoscopic vs. open colectomy. Surg Endosc 2002;16:1420–1425.
46 Zutshi M, Delaney C, Senagore A, Mekhail N, Lewis B, Connor J, Fazio V: Randomized controlled trial comparing the controlled rehabilitation with early ambulation and diet pathway versus the controlled rehabilitation with early ambulation and diet with preemptive epidural anesthesia/analgesia after laparotomy and intestinal resection. Am J Surg 2005;189:268–272.
47 Larach S, Patankar S, Ferrara A, Williamson P, Perozo S, Lord A: Complications of laparoscopic colorectal surgery: analysis and comparison of early vs. latter experience. Dis Colon Rectum 1997;40:592–596.
48 Patankar S, Lee W: Current status of laparoscopic resection for colorectal cancer. J Clin Gastroenterol 2004;38:621–627.
49 Wishner J, Baker JJ, Hoffman G, Hubbard G, Gould R, Wophlgemuth S, Ruffin W, Melick C: Laparoscopic-assisted colectomy. The learning curve. Surg Endosc 1995;9:1179–1183.
50 Falk P, Beart RJ, Wexner S, Thorson A, Jagelman D, Lavery I, Johansen O, Fitzgibbons RJ: Laparoscopic colectomy: a critical appraisal. Dis Colon Rectum 1993;36:28–34.
51 Fleshman J, Nelson H, Peters W, Kim H, Larach S, Boorse R, Ambroze W, Leggett P, et al: Early results of laparoscopic surgery for colorectal cancer: retrospective analysis of 372 patients treated by Clinical Outcomes of Surgical Therapy (COST) Study Group. Dis Colon Rectum 1996;39:S53–S58.
52 Fleshman J, Wexner S, Anvari M, LaTulippe J, Birnbaum E, Read T, Nogueras J, Weiss E: Laparoscopic vs. open abdominoperineal resection for cancer. Dis Colon Rectum 1999; 42:930–939.
53 Franklin M, Kazantsev B, Abrego D, Diaz E, Balli J, Glass J: Laparoscopic surgery for stage III colon cancer: long-term follow-up. Surg Endosc 2000;14:612–616.
54 Franklin MJ, Rosenthal D, Abrego-Medina D, Dorman J, Glass J, Norem R, Diaz A: Prospective comparison of open vs. laparoscopic colon surgery for carcinoma: five-year results. Dis Colon Rectum 1996;39:S35–S46.
55 Khalili T, Fleshner P, Hiatt J, Sokol T, Manookian C, Tsushima G, Phillips E: Colorectal cancer: comparison of laparoscopic with open approaches. Dis Colon Rectum 1998; 41:832–838.
56 Leung K, Yiu R, Lai P, Lee J, Thung K, Lau W: Laparoscopic-assisted resection of colorectal carcinoma: five-year audit. Dis Colon Rectum 1999;42:327–332.
57 Peters W, Bartels T: Minimally invasive colectomy: are the potential benefits realized? Dis Colon Rectum 1993;36:751–756.
58 Schiedeck T, Schwandner O, Baca I, Baehrlehner E, Konradt J, Kockerling F, Kuthe A, Buerk C, et al: Laparoscopic surgery for the cure of colorectal cancer: results of a German five-centre study. Dis Colon Rectum 2000; 43:1–8.
59 Senagore A, Luchtefeld M, Mackeigan J, Mazier W: Open colectomy versus laparoscopic colectomy: are there differences? Am Surg 1993;59:549–554.
60 Stocchi L, Nelson H: Wound recurrences following laparoscopic-assisted colectomy. Arch Surg 2000;135:948–958.
61 Stocchi L, Nelson H, Young-Fadok T, Larson D, Ilstrup D: Safety and advantages of laparoscopic vs. open colectomy in the elderly: matched-control study. Dis Colon Rectum 2000;43:326–332.
62 Kehlet H, Wilmore D: Multimodal strategies to improve surgical outcome. Am J Surg 2002;183:630–641.
63 Bardram L, Funch-Jensen P, Jensen P, Crawford M, Kehlet H: Recovery after laparoscopic colonic surgery with epidural analgesia, and early oral nutrition and mobilization. Lancet 1995;345:763–764.
64 Wind J, Polle S, Fung Kon Jin P, Dejong C, von Meyenfeldt M, Ubbink D, Gouma D, Bemelman W: Laparoscopy and/or Fast Track Multimodal Management Versus Standard Care (LAFA) study group and the Enhanced Recovery After Surgery (ERAS) group. Systematic review of enhanced recovery programmes in colonic surgery. Br J Surg 2006; 93:800–809.
65 Marusch F, Gastinger I, Schneider C, Scheidbach H, Konradt J, Bruch H, Kohler L, Barlehner E, Kockerling F: Importance of conversion for results obtained with laparoscopic colorectal surgery. Dis Colon Rectum 2001;44:207–216.
66 Gervaz P, Pikarsky A, Utech M, Secic M, Efron M, Belin B, Jain A, Wexner S: Converted laparoscopic surgery. A meta-analysis. Surg Endosc 2001;15:827–832.
67 Pandya S, Murray J, Coller J, Rusin L: Laparoscopic colectomy: indications for conversion to laparotomy. Arch Surg 1999;134:471–475.
68 Marusch F, Gastinger I, Schneider C, Scheidbach H, Konradt J, Bruch H, Kohler L, Barlehner E, Kockerling F: Experience as a factor influencing the indications for laparoscopic colorectal surgery and the results. Surg Endosc 2001;15:116–120.
69 Schwandner O, Schiedeck T, Bruch H: The role of conversion in laparoscopic colorectal surgery. Do predictive factors exist? Surg Endosc 1999;13:151–156.
70 Tekkis P, Senagore A, Delaney C: Conversion rates in laparoscopic colorectal surgery. A predictive model with 1,253 patients. Surg Endosc 2005;19:47–54.
71 Slim K, Pezet D, Riff Y, Clark E, Chipponi J: High morbidity rate after converted laparoscopic colorectal surgery. Br J Surg 1995;82: 1406–1408.
72 Belizon A, Sardinha C, Sher M: Converted laparoscopic colectomy: What are the consequences? Surg Endosc 2006;20:947–951.
73 Moloo H, Mamazza J, Poulin E, Burpee S, Bendavid Y, Klein L, Gregoire R, Schlachta C: Laparoscopic resections for colorectal cancer: does conversion affect survival? Surg Endosc 2004;18:732–735.
74 Schlachta C, Mamazza J, Poulin E, Seshadri P, Cadeddu M, Poulin E: Predicting conversion to open surgery in laparoscopic colorectal resections. A simple clinical model. Surg Endosc 2000;14:1114–1117.
75 Walker K, Bell S, Rickard M, Mehanna D, Dent O, Chapuis P, Bokey E: Anastomotic leakage is predictive of diminished survival after potentially curative resection for colorectal cancer. Ann Surg 2004;240:255–259.
76 Casillas S, Delaney C, Senagore A, Brady K, Fazio V: Does conversion of a laparoscopic colectomy adversely affect patient outcome? Dis Colon Rectum 2004;47:1680–1685.
77 Nelson H, Petrelli N, Carlin A, Couture J, Fleshman J, Guillem J, Ota D, Sargent D: Guidelines 2000 for colon and rectal cancer surgery. J Natl Cancer Inst 2001;93:583–596.
78 Nelson R, Chezmar J, Sugarbaker P, Murray D, Bernardino M: Preoperative localization of focal liver lesions to specific liver segments: utility of CT during arterial portography. Radiology 1990;176:89–84.
79 Stark D, Wittenberg J, Butch R, Ferrucci JJ: Hepatic metastases: randomized, controlled comparison of detection with MR imaging and CT. Radiology 1987;165:399–406.
80 Van Beers B, Gallez B, Pringot J: Contrast-enhanced MR imaging of the liver. Radiology 1997;203:297–306.

81 Foroutani A, Garland A, Beber E, String A, Engle K, Ryan T, Pearl J, Siperstein A: Laparoscopic ultrasound vs. triphasic computed tomography for detecting liver tumors. Arch Surg 2000;135:933–938.
82 Stewart P, Chu J, Kos S, Chapuis P, Bokey E: Intraoperative ultrasound for the detection of hepatic metastases from colorectal cancer. Aust NZ J Surg 1993;63:530–534.
83 Berends F, Kazemier G, Bonjer H, Lange J: Subcutaneous metastases after laparoscopic colectomy. Lancet 1994;344:358.
84 Fingerhut A, Millat B, Lointier P, Hay J: Is laparoscopic colonic resection for carcinoma feasible and safe? A French collective experience. Dig Dis 1995;12:280–283.
85 Lord S, Larach S, Ferrara A, Williamson P, Lago C, Lube M: Laparoscopic resections for colorectal carcinoma: a three-year experience. Dis Colon Rectum 1996;39:148–154.
86 Patankar S, Larach S, Ferrara A, Williamson P, Gallagher J, DeJesus S, Narayanan S: Prospective comparison of laparoscopic vs. open resections for colorectal adenocarcinoma over a ten-year period. Dis Colon Rectum 2003;46:601–611.
87 Pearlstone D, Mansfield P, Curley S, Cook P, Feig B: Laparoscopy in 533 patients with abdominal malignancy. Surgery 1999;125:67–72.
88 Poulin E, Mamazza J, Schlachta C, Gregoire R, Roy N: Laparoscopic resection does not adversely affect early survival curves in patients undergoing surgery for colorectal adenocarcinoma. Ann Surg 1999;229:487–492.
89 Vukasin P, Ortega A, Greene F, Steele G, Simons A, Anthone G, Weston L, Beart RJ: Wound recurrence following laparoscopic colon cancer resection: results of the American Society of Colon and Rectal Surgeons Laparoscopic Registry. Dis Colon Rectum 1996;39:S20–S23.
90 Guillou P, Darzi A, Monson J: Experience with laparoscopic colorectal surgery for malignant disease. Surg Oncol 1993;2:43–49.
91 Hughes E, McDermott F, Polglase A, Johnson W: Tumor recurrence in the abdominal wall scar tissue after large-bowel cancer surgery. Dis Colon Rectum 1983;26:571–572.
92 Reilly W, Nelson H, Schroeder G, Wieand H, Bolton J, O'Connell M: Wound recurrence following conventional treatment of colorectal cancer: a rare but perhaps underestimated problem. Dis Colon Rectum 1996;39:200–207.
93 Ceulemans R, Herni M, Dutson E, Leroy J, Marescaux J: Open versus laparoscopy-assisted colectomy. Lancet 2003;361:73–74.
94 Evrard S, Mathoulin-Pelissier S, Kramar A: Open versus laparoscopy-assisted colectomy. Lancet 2003;361:73.
95 Lehnert T, Abel U, Kienle P, Hinz U: Open versus laparoscopy-assisted colectomy. Lancet 2003;361:74.
96 Lacy A, Delgado S, Castells A, Pique J: Open versus laparoscopy-assisted colectomy. Lancet 2003;381:75–76.
97 Lacy A, Garcia-Valdecasas J, Delgado S, Grande L, Fuster J, Tabet J, Ramos C, Pique J, Cifuentes A, Visa J: Postoperative complications of laparoscopic-assisted colectomy. Surg Endosc 1997;11:119–122.
98 Tinmouth J, Tomlinson G: Laparoscopically-assisted versus open colectomy for colon cancer. N Eng J Med 2004;351:933.
99 Bokey E, Moore J, Chapuis P, Newland R: Morbidity and mortality following laparoscopic-assisted right hemicolectomy for cancer. Dis Colon Rectum 1996;39:S24–S28.
100 Geis W, Coletta A, Verdeja J, Plasencia G, Ojogho O, Jacobs M: Sequential psychomotor skills development in laparoscopic colon surgery. Arch Surg 1994;129:206–212.
101 Tekkis P, Senagore A, Delaney C, Fazio V: Evaluation of the learning curve in laparoscopic colorectal surgery: comparison of right-sided and left-sided resections. Ann Surg 2005;242:83–91.
102 Philipson B, Bokey E, Moore J, Chapuis P, Bagge E: Cost of open versus laparoscopically-assisted right hemicolectomy for cancer. World J Surg 1997;21:214–217.
103 Bouvet M, Mansfield P, Skibber J, Curley S, Ellis L, Giacco G, Madary A, Ota D, Feig B: Clinical, pathologic, and economic parameters of laparoscopic colon resection for cancer. Am J Surg 1999;176:554–558.
104 Delaney C, Kiran R, Senagore A, Brady K, Fazio V: Case-matched comparison of clinical and financial outcome after laparoscopic or open colorectal surgery. Ann Surg 2003;238:67–72.
105 Braga M, Vignali A, Zuliani W, Frasson M, Di Serio C, Di Carlo V: Laparoscopic versus open colorectal surgery: cost-benefit analysis in a single-center randomized trial. Ann Surg 2005;242:890–895.
106 Salloum R, Bulter D, Schwartz S: Economic evaluation of minimally invasive colectomy. J Am Coll Surg 2006;202:269–274.
107 Janson M: Laparoscopic and Open Surgery for Colon Cancer. Studies on Costs and Health-Related Quality of Life. Stockholm, Karolinska Institutet, 2006.
108 Milsom J, Kim H, Hammerhofer K, Fazio V: Laparoscopic colorectal cancer surgery for palliation. Dis Colon Rectum 2000;43:1512–1516.
109 Koea J, Guillem J, Conlon K, Minsky B, Saltz L, Cohen A: Role of laparoscopy in the initial multimodality management of patients with near-obstructing rectal cancer. J Gastrointest Surg 2000;4:105–108.
110 Hodgson N, Malthaner R, Ostbye T: The search for an ideal method of abdominal fascial closure: a meta-analysis. Ann Surg 2000;231:436–442.
111 Scott D, Jones D: Abdominal wall defects; in Norton J, Bollinger R, Chang A, Lowry S, Mulvihil S, Pass H, Thompson R (eds): Surgery: Basic Science and Clinical Evidence. New York, Springer, 2001, pp 813–819.
112 Mayol J, Garcia-Aguilar J, Ortiz-Oshiro E, De-Diego Carmona J, Fernandez-Represa J: Risks of the minimal access approach for laparoscopic surgery: multivariate analysis of morbidity related to umbilical trocar insertion. World J Surg 1997;21:529–533.
113 Tonouchi H, Ohmori Y, Kobayashi M, Kusunoki M: Trocar site hernia. Arch Surg 2004;139:1248–1256.
114 Lumley J, Stitz R, Stevenson A, Fielding G, Luck A: Laparoscopic colorectal surgery for cancer: intermediate to long-term outcomes. Dis Colon Rectum 2002;45:867–872.
115 Marcello P, Roberts P, Rusin L, Holubkov R, Schoetz D: Vascular pedicle ligation techniques during laparoscopic colectomy. A prospective randomized trial. Surg Endosc 2006;20:263–269.
116 Morino M, Rimonda R, Allaix M, Giraudo G, Garrone C: Ultrasonic versus standard electric dissection in laparoscopic colorectal surgery: a prospective randomized clinical trial. Ann Surg 2005;242:897–901.
117 Takada M, Ichihara T, Kuroda Y: Comparative study of electrothermal bipolar vessel sealer and ultrasonic coagulating shears in laparoscopic colectomy. Surg Endosc 2005;19:226–228.
118 Targarona E, Balague C, Marin J, Neto R, Martinez C, Garriga J, Trias M: Energy sources for laparoscopic colectomy: a prospective randomized comparison of conventional electrosurgery, bipolar computer-controlled electrosurgery and ultrasonic dissection. Operative outcome and costs analysis. Surg Innov 2005;12:339–344.

Review Article

Digestive Diseases

Dig Dis 2007;25:44–50
DOI: 10.1159/000099169

Definition of Total Mesorectal Excision, Including the Perineal Phase: Technical Considerations

Klaas Havenga[a] Irene Grossmann[a] Marco DeRuiter[b] Theo Wiggers[a]

[a]Department of Surgery, University Medical Center Groningen, and [b]Department of Embryology and Anatomy, Leiden University Medical Center, Leiden, The Netherlands

Key Words

Mesorectal excision, anatomical details · Total mesorectal excision · Total mesorectal excision, perineal phase · Rectal surgery, anatomy

Abstract

Background: Total mesorectal excision (TME) has contributed to a decline in local recurrence. The operation is difficult because of the complicated anatomy of the pelvis and the narrow spaces in the pelvis. We review the anatomy related to TME and we present our surgical technique. ***Anatomy:*** The pelvis can be divided into a parietal compartment and a visceral compartment. Both compartments are covered by a fascial layer: the parietal and the visceral fascia. A space between these fascial layers can be opened by dividing loose areolar tissue. The pelvic autonomic nerves consist of the sympathetic hypogastric nerve and the parasympathetic sacral splanchnic nerve. At the pelvic sidewall these nerves join in the inferior hypogastric plexus. ***Surgery:*** We present our surgical technique based on careful dissection under direct vision and describe our approach to abdominoperineal resection in the knee-chest position. This position enables en bloc resection of the levator ani muscle with the mesorectum, preventing positive circumferential margins in distal rectal tumor. ***Conclusion:*** TME is a difficult and challenging operation. Continuous attention to surgical technique and anatomy is important to keep up the high standards of contemporary rectal surgery.

Introduction

The mesorectum is the fatty tissue envelop of the rectum, containing blood and lymph vessels, lymph nodes and autonomic nerves. The majority of patients with rectal cancer present with disease confined to the mesorectal package. Intact removal of this package is necessary to obtain cure for the disease.

This concept of total mesorectal excision (TME) in rectal cancer surgery was introduced by Heald [1] in 1979. The technique of TME is based on sharp dissection under direct vision following the lipoma-like surface of the mesorectum. This plane is usually avascular and enables identification and preservation of the autonomic nerve plexus [2]. In their landmark paper in the *Lancet* (1993), MacFarlane et al. [3] analyzed the results of the first 13 years of experience with TME presenting a hitherto unprecedented local recurrence rate of 4%. These results were backed up by the personal series of Enker et al. [4] who presented a 7.4% local recurrence rate in 1995. In Japan, Moriya et al. [5] published excellent local control (9.3%) after TME combined with extended lymphadenectomy.

In the mid 1990s, TME was introduced in The Netherlands and in Scandinavia by workshops, live video demonstrations of operations and tutoring of individual surgeons. In the Dutch TME trial, local recurrence after a median follow-up of 2 years was reduced to 2.4% after 5 × 5 Gy radiation therapy and TME and to 8.2% after

KARGER

Fax +41 61 306 12 34
E-Mail karger@karger.ch
www.karger.com

0257–2753/07/0251–0044$23.50/0

Accessible online at:
www.karger.com/ddi

Klaas Havenga, MD, PhD
University Medical Center Groningen
Department of Surgery, PO Box 30.001
NL–9700 RB Groningen (The Netherlands)
Tel. +31 50 361 2283, Fax +31 50 361 4873, E-Mail k.havenga@chir.umcg.nl

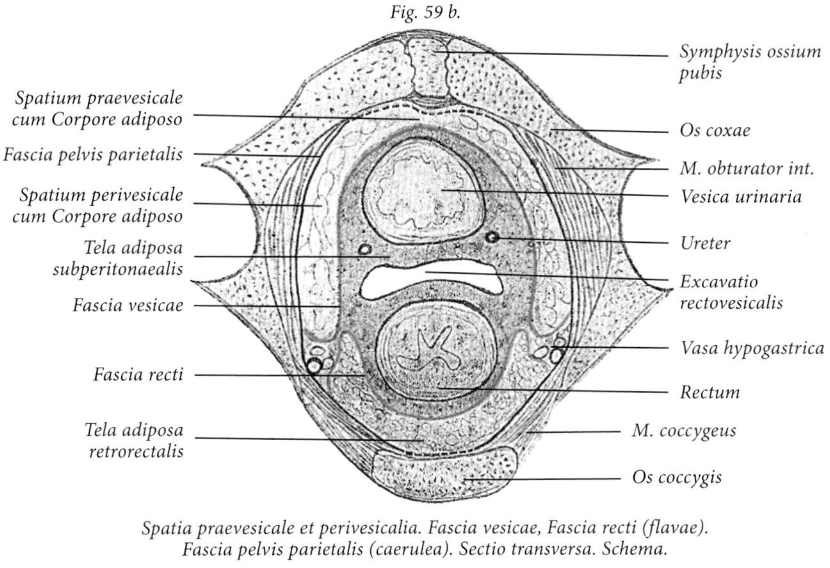

Fig. 1. Transverse section of the pelvis demonstrating the prevesical and retrorectal space. Note the exaggerated width of the loose areolar tissue layer [from W. Waldeyer: Das Becken. Bonn, Friedrich Cohen, 1899, fig. 59b, p. 227].

TME alone [6]. Compared to historical controls, local recurrence was reduced from 28 to 8% after introduction of TME in Norway [7].

Autonomic nerve preservation seems to be successful in maintaining sexual function, although abdominoperineal resection and older age are associated with an increased likelihood on impotence [8]. Identification of the pelvic autonomic nerves and nerve plexus is difficult however, as the nerves are small and visibility in the pelvis is limited, especially in typical obese Western males.

Several reports indicate poor results of abdominoperineal resection for distal rectal tumors [9–11]. In the Dutch TME study, abdominoperineal resection was associated with a higher positive circumferential margin (APR 30.4%, LAR 10.7%). It has been proposed that a wider 'cylindrical' resection should be performed in the case of APR to overcome this problem [12].

TME is a difficult operation because of the complicated anatomy with multiple possible surgical dissection planes and the narrow spaces in the pelvis. There is a definite need for continuous education in rectal cancer surgery to keep up the accomplished high standard of surgery. To contribute to this we review the anatomical details of mesorectal excision in this paper. Subsequently, we will present a detailed description of the operation as we perform it, with special emphasis to the perineal phase.

Anatomy and Embryology

The pelvis may be considered as a two-compartment structure. The outer compartment is the parietal compartment, i.e. the pelvic wall. This compartment consists of the bony and muscular pelvic wall: posteriorly the sacrum and coccyx, the piriformis muscle and coccygeal muscle; inferiorly the levator ani muscle; anteriorly the pubic and iliac bone and the obturator muscle. The inner compartment is the visceral compartment. This compartment consists of the rectum, the bladder and the uterus and vagina in females or the prostate and seminal vesicles in male. The parietal compartment is covered with a parietal fascia. This fascia is continuous with the fascia of the piriformis muscle, the coccygeal muscle and the levator ani muscle. On the sacrum, the parietal fascia is at some places fixed to or identical to the periosteum, at other places a presacral venous plexus is found under the parietal fascia.

The visceral compartment is enveloped in the visceral fascia. Posteriorly the visceral fascia covers the mesorectum, forming its shiny outer surface. The visceral fascia is connected with a layer of loose areolar tissue which can be easily divided. Division of this loose areolar tissue opens the space of Retzius anteriorly (between bladder and pubic bone). Posteriorly, division of this layer of areolar tissue opens the retrorectal space, in surgical literature this dissection plane is referred to as the holy plane

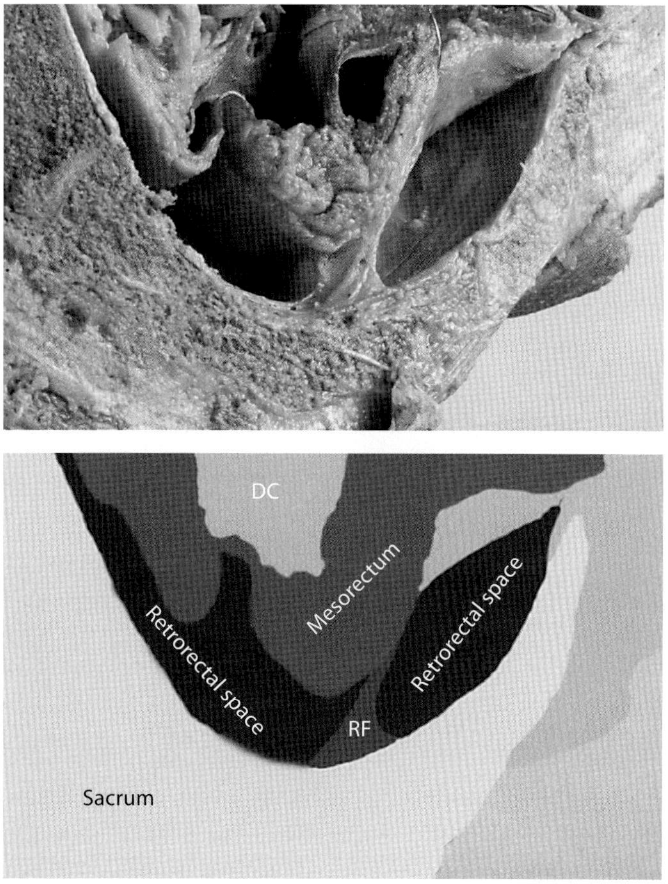

Fig. 2. Midsagittal section of a male pelvis. Detail of the rectosacral fascia (RF). DC = Douglas' cavity.

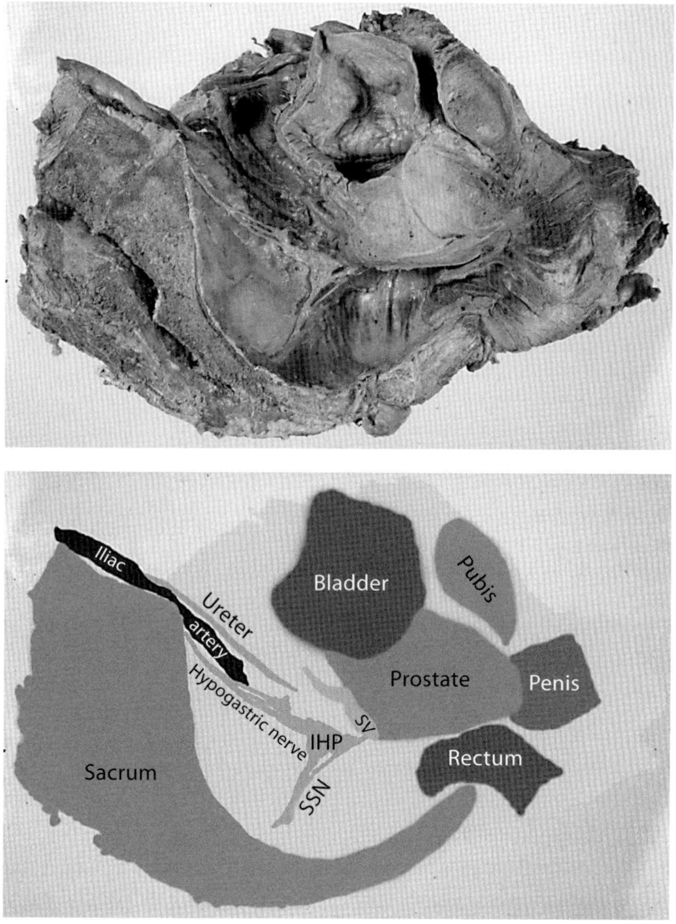

Fig. 3. Midsagittal section of a male pelvis. The mesorectum is removed. IHP = Inferior hypogastric plexus; SSN = sacral splanchnic nerve; SV = seminal vesicle.

[13] or the TME plane. Laterally, the visceral fascia adheres to the pelvic side wall in a zone over and along the iliac vessels (fig. 1).

For a correct understanding of the visceral fascia of the rectum and the organization of the mesorectum, knowledge of the embryology is helpful. Fritsch [14, 15] demonstrated that the mesorectum and the visceral fascia originate from a layer of dense mesenchyme found in 9- to 12-week-old fetuses. In a later stage (13–20 weeks of age) this mesenchyme has organized itself in circular and semicircular lamellae of connective tissue. In the 21- to 38-week-old fetus adipose tissue develops within these connective tissue layers. The most external lamellae however remain dense and may be regarded as the visceral fascia.

Boundaries of the Retrorectal Space. As mentioned above, the visceral fascia adheres to the pelvic sidewall in a zone overlying the iliac vessels. As the iliac vessels originate from the aortic bifurcation, this defines the cranial boundary of the retrorectal space. Caudally, the retrorectal space extends to the anus. A double layer of the visceral fascia is found at the level of S3 where a posterior leaf of the visceral fascia forms a firm attachment to sacrum. This fascia is called the retrorectal fascia (fig. 2). In many publications this fascia is identified as Waldeyer's fascia. In Waldeyer's book 'Das Becken' (The Pelvis), this fascia is not mentioned however.

Pelvic Autonomic Nerves (fig. 3). The pelvic autonomic nerves have a sympathetic and a parasympathetic component. The sympathetic component originates from ventral roots of L2 and L3 to form a preaortic superior hypogastric plexus. At the level of the aortic bifurcation, or a little lower at the level of the promontory, this superior hypogastric plexus forms two hypogastric nerves

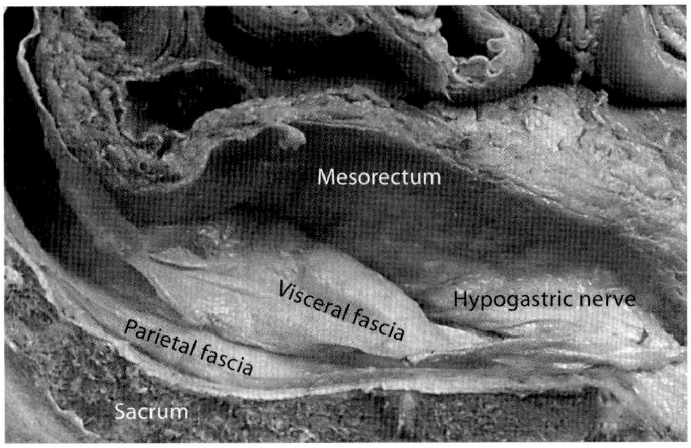

Fig. 4. Sagittal hemisection of a male pelvis. View from above to the right side of the pelvis. The parietal fascia and the visceral fascia are demonstrated. The hypogastric nerve is situated within the outer perimeter of the mesorectum, ventral to the visceral fascia.

which run laterally and caudally, parallel to the ureter. At the level of the promontory these hypogastric nerves are usually situated 1 cm lateral to the midline and 2 cm medial to the ureter. The hypogastric nerve is situated within the periphery of the mesorectum: the visceral fascia of the mesorectum can be demonstrated dorsal to the nerve (fig. 4).

The parasympathetic sacral splanchnic nerves (SSNs) originate from the roots of S3 and S4 and sometimes from S2. The S3 root is usually the largest. These SSNs enter the pelvis through their respective sacral foramen. The SSNs remain in the parietal compartment of the pelvis, posterior to the parietal fascia to a point about 3 cm lateral to the foramen. Here they penetrate the parietal fascia and continue laterally and caudally in the visceral compartment, close to the pelvic side wall, where they meet the hypogastric nerve to form the inferior hypogastric plexus.

Surgical Considerations

In open surgery, rectal resection requires optimal exposure. An incision is made from the pubic bone to approximately 5 cm cranial of the umbilicus. After careful inspection of the abdominal cavity and the liver, a self-retaining retractor is installed. Dissection is started with the incision of the line of Toldt, mobilizing the sigmoid colon from Toldt's fascia. Throughout the operation, careful dissection based on traction and countertraction is performed. Dissection itself is performed by diathermia or scissors. If performed carefully, this mobilization of the sigmoid colon does not breach Toldt's fascia which covers the ureter and the spermatic or ovarian vessels. As the left ureter can be clearly identified this way, we do not advocate routine looping of the ureter.

The mesosigmoid is inspected and transected at a level usually just distal to the first or second sigmoidal artery. The sigmoid is divided with a linear stapler/cutter. Now the peritoneum is opened just medial to the right iliac artery. Careful dissection of the loose areolar tissue at the level of the promontory just posterior to the superior rectal artery mobilizes the most cranial mesorectum while preserving the superior hypogastric plexus and nervus. It is possible to extend the dissection cranially to include the base of the inferior mesenteric artery (IMA) in the specimen. The IMA should be divided leaving a small stump of approximately 1 cm in order to avoid damage to the superior hypogastric plexus at this level. The inferior mesenteric vein is divided at the same level.

In case of a low anastomosis, care has to be given to make a well-circulated loop of descending colon and/or sigmoid with enough length to reach the distal stump without tension. In many cases the sigmoid arteries are too short to allow the colon to reach the rectal stump. We divide the superior rectal artery at its origin from the IMA, and we divide the IMA between its origin from the aorta and the confluens of left colic artery and sigmoid artery. In this way an extra level of collateral circulation to the colon loop is preserved, beside the marginal artery. Furthermore, the length of the colon loop is not limited by a rather short sigmoid artery. Mobilization of the splenic flexure is still often necessary in these cases however.

After the sigmoid colon loop is put behind a blade of the self-retaining retractor, the distal sigmoid/rectal loop is gently lifted ventrally and caudally. Now both hypogastric nerves should be identified. Careful dissection of the hypogastric nerves is performed, taking the mesorectum away from the nerves but leaving the nerves on the sacrum. As the dissection continues downward, the left and right hypogastric nerves diverge. Usually a fascial layer can be divided in the space between the left and right hypogastric nerve. Dividing this fascial layer opens the plane between the most peripheric layer of the mesorectum (the visceral fascia) and the parietal fascia. A step in level of dissection is made at this point at the hypogastric nerve as the hypogastric nerve is located just inside the visceral fascia of the mesorectum. This step is made close to the lateral boundary of the retrorectal space and has usually no clinical significance. When the tumor is close to the hypogastric nerve, it is obvious that resection of the tumor necessitates the sacrifice of the hypogastric nerve. Furthermore, when a total pelvic exenteration is planned, the resection plane is posterior to both hypogastric nerves, extending to the plane posterior to the ureter at the level of the common iliac artery, as preservation of the pelvic autonomic nerves is no issue in these cases.

As the dissection continues downward the retrorectal space is opened. Some small veins cross this space and should be coagulated. Exposure in this plane can be facilitated by using a St Mark's retractor. In most cases, except for slim female patients, exposure gets poor after some progress in this plane. Attention will be shifted to the ventral plane. The incision in the peritoneum is extended ventrally and medially. In male patients the peritoneum is divided some centimeters cranial to the peritoneal reflection on the seminal vesicles. In female patients a corresponding location is found on the posterior fornix of the vagina. To obtain exposure of this area in female patients, it is helpful to elevate the uterus to the abdominal wall with a stitch. Stretching the vagina with a sponge-holding forceps is helpful to identify the posterior fornix. In case of a large uterus, it may be necessary to perform a hysterectomy in order to obtain exposure.

After opening the peritoneum the seminal vesicles in males or the posterior vaginal wall in females is identified. Dissection is continued on the seminal vesicles or posterior vaginal wall. In this way, Denonvilliers' fascia is retained to the specimen as advised by Heald et al. [16]. After developing the anterior plane for some distance, posterior exposure is improved as the mesorectum can be lifted somewhat more from the pelvis. It is frequently necessary or helpful to shift the focus of dissection from time to time during the operation.

The posterior dissection continues to expose the parietal fascia overlying the piriformis muscle. Just caudal to the piriformis muscle the third SSN is located. The SSN originates from the sacral foramen, it enters the pelvis 2–3 cm from the midline. As the SSN runs laterally, it is covered by parietal fascia for another 3 cm before entering a double layer of visceral fascia. Visible identification of the SSN may be difficult because of limited vision into the operating field. If the correct plane in the retrorectal space is followed, damage to the SSNs is unlikely in the median 8 cm of the sacrum, because of the location of the SSN posterior to the parietal fascia. In many cases, it is possible to continue the posterior dissection at this point before the lateral dissection is undertaken. At the level of S3 the rectosacral fascia is encountered. Sharp division of this fascia is necessary in order to prevent a shift of the dissection into the distal mesorectal tissue. Avulsion of the rectosacral fascia from the sacrum may cause serious bleeding from the presacral venous plexus. Distal to the rectosacral fascia the sacrum curves forward towards the anus. Opening of the retrorectal space at this point requires cutting of rather strong, fibrous adhesions. Because of the depth of the dissection, extended diathermia may be too short: long scissors are more practical in that case. We use combined aspiration-illumination devices to facilitate this deep dissection.

Now the lateral dissection may be started. Medial and anterior traction of the specimen allows dissection over the piriformis muscle and on the hypogastric nerve. The hypogastric nerve leads to the inferior hypogastric plexus on the pelvic side wall, just lateral and dorsal to the seminal vesicles in males. The SSN also leads to the inferior hypogastric plexus. At the inferior hypogastric plexus, autonomic nerve branches enter the mesorectum. These branches should be divided in case of TME. (In case of posterior rectopexy division of the autonomic branches to the mesorectum will cause obstipation.) It is easy to dissect into the inferior hypogastric plexus as median traction on the specimen will displace this plexus medial. If tumor is suspected close to the inferior hypogastric plexus (by means of palpation or MRI scan), or if a total pelvic exenteration is performed, a plane lateral to the inferior hypogastric plexus can be chosen.

At this point in the operation, the mesorectum is mobilized to an imaginary transverse ring extending to the distal sacrum posteriorly, the prostate or posterior vaginal wall ventrally and distal to the SSNs and inferior hypogastric plexus laterally. Continuation of the dissection posteriorly and laterally opens the plane between the mesorectum and coccygeal muscle and levator ani muscle. In the case of a low anterior resection, this plane will be dissected until the distal rectum is reached, just above the anus. The mesorectal fatty layer covering the distal rectum thins out to a point it is no longer existent. Here the rectum may be divided using a right angle stapler or right angle stapler/cutter. The specimen is now delivered in the case of a low anterior resection.

If the tumor is located in the proximal rectum, above the peritoneal reflection, the rectum may be divided at a higher point, at least 5 cm below the tumor. This will put the anastomosis at a greater distance from the anus which will reduce the likelihood of incontinence or anastomotic leakage.

If the tumor is located in the distal third of the rectum, the circumferential margin to the mesorectal surface is small, especially in T3 tumors. In our opinion it is not wise to perform a low anterior resection in these cases. Instead, we perform an abdominoperineal resection with en bloc resection of the levator ani muscle. After the anterior resection has reached the transverse line to the distal sacrum and prostate as described above, we finish the abdominal phase. We routinely perform an omentoplasty with the stalk on the right gastroepiploic vessels. The omentoplasty is brought to the pelvis through a small hole in the transverse mesocolon. A colostomy on the descending colon or sigmoid is made and the abdomen is closed.

We then turn the patient in the knee-chest position. Special care has to be given to this positioning. Gravity will cause maximal flexion of the knees, causing damage. To prevent this we put a roll under the upper legs. The operation table is put to some degrees of anti-Trendelenburg to balance the patient in a way that most of the weight is transferred to the knees. The chest is supported with a large, firm but soft roll. In this way the abdomen is hanging freely, facilitating ventilation.

Performing the perineal phase in the knee-chest position instead of the standard position in stirrups has several advantages: (a) exposure to the operative field is better; (b) hydrostatic venous pressure is lower, reducing bleeding; (c) assistance and tutoring is feasible, and (d) gravity will pull the perineum downwards, flattening the pelvic floor.

The perineal phase is started with closure of the anus with a strong pursestring stitch. The perineal skin is incised in an ellipse extending to the perineum ventrally, and extending some centimeters lateral to the anus. Dorsally the incision extends to below the coccyx. In selected cases we extend this incision to include the coccyx or distal sacrum. Ventrally, the posterior vaginal wall in female patients may be included in the resection. The ischiorectal fat is then divided using diathermia. Some branches of the inferior rectal artery and vein are encountered. Continuing this dissection will expose the inferior-outer surface of the levator ani muscle and its insertion to the obturator muscle. Ventrally the perineal muscle will be divided. This will expose the bulbus of the penis in male patients or the posterior vaginal wall in female patients. In male patients the ventral plane leads from the bulbus to the urethra. A transurethral catheter is helpful to identify the urethra by palpation. After dissecting the urethra it may be difficult to continue in the correct plane on the prostate because of a sharp angle in the dissection plane. As dissection on the bulbus, urethra and prostate is carried out, the left and right levator muscle stands out as vertical columns which can be divided. Step by step the prostate is dissected and the levator is divided. On the posterior side the dissection plane of the laparotomy will be met. In some cases some upward dissection has to be made to reach this plane. Some authors advocate entering the retrorectal plane below the tip of the coccyx. The levator ani muscle can then be divided by hooking this muscle by a finger. We believe this maneuver carries the risk of exposing the distal mesorectal surface and possibly the tumor. Our technique of the perineal phase ensures that the levator ani muscle is resected en bloc with the specimen, avoiding a positive margin in distal T3 tumors because of a thin distal mesorectal layer.

The specimen can now be removed. As the levator is completely resected, the perineal wound presents as a large defect in the pelvic floor. We use the omentoplasty to close this perineal defect. If it is not possible to make an omentoplasty, a rectus abdominus flap will be used.

After fixating the omentoplasty or rectus flap in the perineal defect the subcutaneous fascia is approximated. Finally, the skin is closed with interrupted sutures.

Conclusion

TME for rectal cancer is a difficult and challenging operation. Detailed knowledge of the anatomy is of crucial importance to perform this operation. We presented our technique of the operation. We would invite others to present their technical approach to the operation. It is important to discuss and study surgical techniques to maintain surgical quality at a high level. It is the patient who will benefit by a reduced risk of local recurrence.

References

1 Heald RJ: A new approach to rectal cancer. Br J Hosp Med 1979;22:277–281.
2 Heald RJ, Husband EM, Ryall RD: The mesorectum in rectal cancer surgery – the clue to pelvic recurrence? Br J Surg 1982;69:613–616.
3 MacFarlane JK, Ryall RD, Heald RJ: Mesorectal excision for rectal cancer. Lancet 1993; 341:457–460.
4 Enker WE, Thaler HT, Cranor ML, Polyak T: Total mesorectal excision in the operative treatment of carcinoma of the rectum. J Am Coll Surg 1995;181:335–346.
5 Moriya Y, Sugihara K, Akasu T, Fujita S: Importance of extended lymphadenectomy with lateral node dissection for advanced lower rectal cancer. World J Surg 1997;21: 728–732.
6 Kapiteijn E, Marijnen CA, Nagtegaal ID, Putter H, Steup WH, Wiggers T, et al: Preoperative radiotherapy combined with total mesorectal excision for resectable rectal cancer. N Engl J Med 2001;345:638–646.
7 Wibe A, Eriksen MT, Syse A, Myrvold HE, Soreide O: Total mesorectal excision for rectal cancer – what can be achieved by a national audit? Colorectal Dis 2003;5:471–477.
8 Havenga K, Enker WE, McDermott K, Cohen AM, Minsky BD, Guillem J: Male and female sexual and urinary function after total mesorectal excision with autonomic nerve preservation for carcinoma of the rectum. J Am Coll Surg 1996;182:495–502.
9 Law WL, Chu KW: Abdominoperineal resection is associated with poor oncological outcome. Br J Surg 2004;91:1493–1499.
10 Nagtegaal ID, van de Velde CJ, Marijnen CA, van Krieken JH, Quirke P: Low rectal cancer: a call for a change of approach in abdominoperineal resection. J Clin Oncol 2005;23: 9257–9264.
11 Marr R, Birbeck K, Garvican J, Macklin CP, Tiffin NJ, Parsons WJ, et al: The modern abdominoperineal excision: the next challenge after total mesorectal excision. Ann Surg 2005;242:74–82.
12 Daniels IR, Strassburg J, Moran BJ: The need for future surgical low rectal cancer studies. Colorectal Dis 2006;8(suppl 3):25–29.
13 Heald RJ: The 'holy plane' of rectal surgery. J R Soc Med 1988;81:503–508.
14 Fritsch H: Development of the rectal fascia (in German). Anat Anz 1990;170:273–280.
15 Fritsch H: Development and organization of the pelvic connective tissue in the human fetus. Ann Anat 1993;175:531–539.
16 Heald RJ, Moran BJ, Brown G, Daniels IR: Optimal total mesorectal excision for rectal cancer is by dissection in front of Denonvilliers' fascia. Br J Surg 2004;91:121–123.

Review Article

Digestive Diseases

Dig Dis 2007;25:51–55
DOI: 10.1159/000099170

Role of Total Mesorectal Excision and of Circumferential Resection Margin in Local Recurrence and Survival of Patients with Rectal Carcinoma

Maria Tzardi

Department of Pathology, University Hospital, Heraklion, Greece

Key Words

Circumferential resection margin · Rectal cancer, histological findings · Rectal cancer, prognostic factors · Rectal carcinoma · Total mesorectal excision

Abstract

Rectal cancer is a common disease with poor prognosis because of local recurrence and metastases. Local recurrence arises mainly as a result of incomplete surgical resection. Evaluation of completeness of the mesorectum provides significant information about prognosis. Total mesorectal excision (TME) has become the surgical treatment of choice for rectal cancer because adopting the principles of TME achieves very low local recurrence rates. The adoption of the TME principles along with the estimation of the circumferential resection margin on the non-peritonealized surface of the resected rectal specimen are the most important predictors of local recurrence.

Introduction

Rectal cancer is a common disease with poor prognosis because of local recurrence and metastases. A number of prognostic factors have been shown to be related to the survival of patients with rectal cancer. Histological grade and type of tumor, vascular and perineural invasion, TNM stage, tumor-specific molecular features and microsatellite instability have prognostic value in rectal cancer. In recent years, histological findings such as the completeness of the total mesorectal resection and the proximity of the tumor to the circumferential resection margin (CRM) have had a strong prognostic value of both local recurrence and survival.

Total Mesorectal Excision

Local recurrence arises mainly as a result of incomplete surgical resection. Mesorectal tissue seems to be an ideal substrate for the spreading of tumor. In rectal cancer, local recurrence is present in the absence of distant metastases and this model is different from that in colon cancer in which the local recurrence is often present with distant metastases [1]. Heald and Ryal [2] first proposed that radical surgery for rectal cancer should include complete resection of the mesorectum. The mesorectum consists of the rectum and the surrounding fat tissue with the perirectal lymph nodes and is enveloped by a thin fascia.

In the past, the rate of local recurrence was as high as 20–50% [2, 3]. According to different studies, the risk of local recurrence ranged from 2.3 to 28 times in cases with spread of tumor to the mesorectum [4]. Studies showed

KARGER

Fax +41 61 306 12 34
E-Mail karger@karger.ch
www.karger.com

0257–2753/07/0251–0051$23.50/0

Accessible online at:
www.karger.com/ddi

Maria Tzardi
Department of Pathology, University Hospital of Heraklion
GR–71110 Heraklion (Greece)
E-Mail tzardi_maria@yahoo.co.uk

that the evaluation of completeness of the mesorectum provides significant information about the prognosis.

Macroscopic examination of the mesorectal surface helps us evaluate the quality of the surgical specimen. Mesorectal defects are classified into three categories: (a) *complete:* mesorectum is intact, smooth with only minor irregularities without defect >5 mm; (b) *moderate:* moderate bulk to mesorectum but irregularity of the mesorectal surface; muscularis propria is not visible with the exception of the area of insertion of levator muscles, and (c) *incomplete:* little bulk to mesorectum with defects down into muscularis propria [1, 5–7].

There is also a grading system used to determine the completeness of the mesorectal excision in which grade 1 indicates incomplete resection, grade 2 nearly complete, and grade 3 complete resection [7–9].

Nagtegaal and van Krieken [6] showed that patients with an incomplete mesorectum have a higher risk of recurrence (36%) than those with complete mesorectum (20%). Several studies have proved that total mesorectal excision (TME) has reduced the local recurrence rates. Heald and Ryal [2] showed that after TME the local recurrence rate was reduced from 30–40% to 5–15%. Arbman et al. [10] have shown that adopting the technique of TME can result in a 20% improvement in the 4-year survival rate, and the Norwegian Rectal Cancer Group [11] showed a greater improvement.

Sometimes there is a disagreement between the surgeon and pathologist, or there cannot be certainty about the completeness of the mesorectum. Martling et al. [12] showed that when the surgeon or pathologist were uncertain or there was a disagreement about the completeness of the mesorectum, the risk of recurrence was similar to that of incomplete resection.

In the literature there are studies which focus on the difference of TME between tumors which are located at ≤6 cm from the anal verge and tumors at >6 cm from the anal verge. They showed that low rectal tumors have a higher rate of recurrence than the tumors at >6 cm and they consider the unresected positive lateral lymph nodes as a possible explanation [13, 14]. Only a Japanese group [14] have performed lateral node dissection after en bloc resection of the rectum, the mesorectum with visceral pelvic fascia and the lateral sidewall structures including the pelvic nerve plexuses. They consider that patients with lateral nodal involvement must have a lateral dissection, even if their results are not based on randomized studies.

The position of the tumor in the circumference of the rectum probably has a clinical value. The results from studies focusing on the position of the tumor are contradictory. A study showed that the circumferential position of the tumor had a worse prognosis than others and anteriorly positioned tumors had a significantly higher survival rate [15]. Another study of 401 patients with rectal cancer showed no difference in the rate of recurrence and the survival based on the position of the tumor. The same study showed that anteriorly placed tumors tend to be more advanced and male patients with an anteriorly placed tumor had a higher risk of recurrence than with tumors in another location. The authors consider that the predilection of gender was a result of different surgical treatment [16].

TME has become the surgical treatment of choice for rectal cancer and now there is an accumulation of evidence indicating that surgeons who have adopted the principles of TME can consistently achieve local recurrence rates of 3–10% and an overall survival rate of up to 80% [1, 2, 5–7, 13, 17–20].

Circumferential Resection Margin

After the introduction of TME, the CRM on the non-peritonealized surface of the resected rectal specimen is one of the most important predictors of local recurrence. Quirke et al. [21] were the first to show that the radial or CRM is an important factor for local recurrence. The CRM can be involved by the tumor in various ways, such as direct spread, by tumor emboli in veins, lymphatics or lymph nodes or by tumor deposits discontinuous from the main growth [21–23].

The rectum is covered anteriorly by peritoneum and only in the area below the peritoneal reflection is there a risk of the CRM being involved. The posterior area, which continues up to the sigmoid mesocolon, is at risk of being involved by the tumor not only by direct spread but also with metastatic deposits in lymph nodes. The mesorectum is thinner anteriorly than posteriorly and the risk of a positive resection margin is higher for anteriorly located tumors than in posterior ones.

Microscopic tumor nodules can be observed in the mesorectum. Studies have shown that the presence of widespread microscopic nodules in the mesorectum was present in up to 38.7%. In 25.8% of cases these were detected in the outer part of the mesorectum. Other studies proved that lymph nodes <5 mm in diameter are more often involved by the tumor than bigger ones. Such findings pinpoint the importance of TME [24–26]. The pathologist must differentiate the peritonealized from non-peritonealized surfaces of the resection. If a tumor is detected on the non-peritonealized surface, adjuvant radiotherapy may be appropriate without the dimensions of the tumor to be considered.

Histological examination of the rectal specimen is based on a method described by Quirke et al. [21]. The lateral resection margin of the fresh surgical specimen must be inked. The surgical specimen is opened apart from the tumor area and 2 cm below and above it. The specimen is fixed for 48 h. After fixation the specimen is sliced transversely at 3- to 4-mm intervals, looking for continuous spread and/or discontinuous tumor deposits and for involved lymph node at the CRM [1, 5, 6, 21, 23, 27–29]. The macroscopic CRM is measured with a ruler; the microscopic CRM measurement is done better by using a sheet of graph paper that is photocopied onto a sheet of acetate and cut to size than to using the Vernier scale [5, 23]. The CRM is divided into two categories: an involved (positive) CRM when the tumor extends to within 1 mm of the circumferential margin and an uninvolved (negative) CRM when the distance between the tumor and CRM is >1 mm [21].

Adam et al. [30] and Quirke et al. [21] showed that involvement of the circumferential margin was detected in 25% of specimens for which the surgeon thought the resection was potentially curative and in 36% of all the cases. The frequency of local recurrence was 78% in patients with tumor involvement of the CRM versus 10% in patients without involvement.

Wibe et al. [31] reviewed the rates of overall survival, local recurrence and distant metastasis in 686 patients with known circumferential margins (margin <1 mm) after TME in order to determine the prognostic impact. Overall local recurrence rate was 7%. The local recurrence was significantly higher in patients with a positive resection margin (22%) versus a negative margin (5%). 40% of patients with positive margin developed distant metastasis versus 12% of patients with a negative margin. They concluded that information on the circumferential margin might help in selecting those patients who should receive adjuvant therapy [31, 32].

Another study showed that cases with positive CRMs have a 37% risk of developing distant metastases versus 15% in cases with margins >1 mm. The same study showed a lower survival rate, 70 vs. 90%, in the 2-year follow-up [6].

All the studies in the literature consider a positive CRM to be a distance between tumor and margin of <1 mm. However, in one study the risk of local recurrence was high at 2 mm. In that study, patients with margins ≤2 mm had a risk of 16% local recurrence within 2 years after operation, while, on the other hand, patients with margins >2 mm had a risk of 5.8% [28]. Several studies have focused on CRM and have indicated that the frequency of positive CRM varied between 15 and 48%, and the authors consider that is influenced by the type of surgery performed. Several studies also indicated that the frequency of a positive CRM is higher in abdominoperineal resection than in low anterior resection [21, 23, 33].

The CRM may be involved by the presence of positive lymph nodes. Nagtegaal et al. [20, 28] showed that the local recurrence rate in patients with a positive resection margin due to a positive lymph node in the resection was not different from the local recurrence rates in patients with negative margins. Some authors consider that there are two different subgroups in the category of positive CRMs if it is compared with the R classification (residual tumor) [23, 34]. They consider that there is a group where the tumor extends up to the CRM, corresponding to R1, and a second group where the tumor is observed ≤1 mm to the CRM, corresponding to R0 [23, 34]. Studies have shown that there is a prognostic difference between the two subgroups, for example Birbeck et al. [29] and Nagtegaal et al. [28] indicated that the rate of local recurrence was 55 and 33% respectively for patients with a tumor at the circumferential margin (R1) versus 28 and 8% respectively in patients with a tumor ≤1 mm from the circumferential margin (R0).

Preoperative Staging

Preoperative staging is used to determine the need for neoadjuvant therapy and to choose the optimal surgical treatment. For this reason, a number of imaging methods are used, including endorectal ultrasound, computed tomography scan, magnetic resonance imaging and positron emission tomography (PET scan) [19]. Studies indicate that patients with positive CRM may benefit from preoperative radiotherapy and that preoperative radiation therapy reduces the local recurrence rate from 8.2 to 2.4% [31, 32, 35]. In advanced rectal cancer it is well documented that long-course preoperative therapy and chemoradiotherapy lead to regression of the tumor.

Most of the radiology studies have focused on T and N stage of rectal cancer rather than on CRMs [19, 35–37]. A few have indicated that high-resolution MRI can be used to determine the status of the circumferential margin [35, 38].

Conclusion

Surgeons make all efforts to improve the surgical techniques in order to obtain negative CRMs. The pathology report gives information which can help determine factors that contribute to local recurrence and decide postoperative treatment. The elements of the pathology report consist of completeness of mesorectum, the CRM, type and grade of the carcinoma, the number of positive lymph nodes and vascular invasion. The newer MRI techniques may play a role in determining preoperatively mesorectum and the CRM in order to select patients with a high risk of CRM involvement and for those patients preoperative radiochemotherapy is the treatment of choice. PET scanning may have a role in determining locally advanced tumor response to neoadjuvant chemotherapy.

It is now obvious that to obtain a low rate of local recurrence and to improve the overall survival of patients with rectal cancer, we need close collaboration between surgeons, pathologists, radiologists and oncologists.

References

1 Compton CC: Pathologic prognostic factors in the recurrence of rectal cancer. Clin Colorectal Cancer 2002;2:149–160.
2 Heald RJ, Ryal RD: Recurrence and survival after total mesorectal excision for rectal cancer. Lancet 1986;i:1479–1482.
3 Nilsson E, Gregersen NP, Hartvig B: Carcinoma of the colon and rectum. Acta Chir Scand 1984;150:513–516.
4 Wang C, Zhou ZG, Wang Z, Li L, Zheng YC, Zhao GP, Chen DY, Liu WP: Mesorectal spread and micrometastasis of rectal cancer studied with large slice technique and tissue microarray. J Surg Oncol 2005;91:167–172.
5 The Pathological Aspect of Rectal Cancer. The TME Workshop by the Pelican Cancer Foundation, 2002.
6 Nagtegaal ID, van Krieken JHJM: The role of pathologists in the quality control of diagnosis and treatment of rectal cancer – an overview. Eur J Cancer 2002;38:964–972.
7 Quirke P: Training and quality assurance for rectal cancer: 20 years of data is enough. Lancet Oncol 2003;4:695–702.
8 Quirke P: Limitations of existing system of staging for rectal cancer; in Rectal Cancer Surgery: Optimization, Standardization and Documentation. Berlin, Springer, 1997, vol 63, p 8132.
9 Nagtegaal ID: Pathological aspects of rectal carcinoma. Studies from RT + TME trial; PhD thesis, Nijmegen 2002.
10 Arbman G, Nilsson E, Hallbook O, Siodahl R: Local recurrence following total mesorectal excision for rectal cancer. Br J Surg 1996; 83:375–379.
11 Norwegian Rectal Cancer Group: Total mesorectal excision in Norway: a national rectal cancer project. Dis Colon Rectum 1999;42: A26.
12 Martling A, Singnomklao T, Holm T, Rutqvist LE, Cedermark B: Prognostic significance of both surgical and pathological assessment of curative resection for rectal cancer. Br J Surg 2004;91:1040–1045.
13 Faerden AE, Naimy N, Wiik P, Reiertsen O, Weyessa S, Tronnes S, Norheim Andersen S, Bakka A: Total mesorectal excision for rectal cancer: difference in outcome for low and high rectal cancer. Dis Colon Rectum 2005; 48:2224–2231.
14 Ueno H, Mochizuki H, Hashiguchi Y, Hase K: Prognostic determinants of patient with lateral nodal involvement by rectal cancer. Ann Surgy 2001;234:190–197.
15 Emslie J, Beart R, Mohiuddin M, Marks G: Use of rectal cancer position as a prognostic indicator. Am Surg 1998;64:958–961.
16 Lee SH, Hernandez de Anda E, Finne CO, Madoff RD, Garcia-Aguila J: The effect of circumferential tumor location in clinical outcomes of rectal cancer patients treated with total mesorectal excision. Dis Colon Rectum 2005;48:2249–2257.
17 Martling AL, Holm T, Rutqvist LE, Moran BJ, Heald RJ, Cedermark B, Stockholm Colorectal Cancer Study Group: Effect of a surgical training programme on outcome of rectal cancer in the County of Stockholm. Basingstoke Bowel Cancer Research Project. Lancet 2000;356:93–96.
18 Nesbakkem A, Nygaard K, Westerheim O, Mala T, Lunde OC: Local recurrence after mesorectal excision for rectal cancer. Eur J Surg Oncol 2002;28:126–134.
19 Balch GC, De Meo A, Guillem JG: Modern management of rectal cancer. World J Gastroenterol 2006;12:3186–3195.
20 Nagtegaal ID, van der Velde CJH, van der Worp E, Kapiteijin E, Quirke P: Macroscopic evaluation of rectal cancer resection specimen: clinical significance of the pathologist in quality control. J Clin Oncol 2002;20: 1729–1734.
21 Quirke P, Durdey P, Dixon MF, Williams NS: Local recurrence of rectal adenocarcinoma due to inadequate surgical resection. Lancet 1986;ii:996–999.
22 Quirke P, Dixon MF: The prediction of local recurrence in rectal adenocarcinoma by histopathological examination. Int J Colorect Dis 1988;3:127–131.
23 Hermanek P, Junginger T: The circumferential resection margin in rectal carcinoma surgery. Tech Coloproctol 2005;9:193–200.
24 Wang Z, Zhou ZG, Wang C, Zhao GP, Chen YD, et al: Microscopic spread of low rectal cancer in regions of mesorectum: pathologic assessment with whole-mount sections. World J Gastroenterol 2004;10:2949–2953.
25 Wang C, Zhou ZG, Wang Z, Chen YD, et al: Nodal spread and micrometastasis within mesorectum. World J Gastroenterol 2005;11: 3586–3590.
26 Wang C, Zhou ZG, Wang Z, Zheng Y, et al: Patterns of neoplastic foci and lymph node micrometastasis within mesorectum. Langenbecks Arch Surg 2005;390:312–318.
27 Quirke P, Williams GT: Minimum Dataset for Colorectal Cancer: Histopathology Reports. London, Royal College of Pathologists, 2004.
28 Nagtegaal ID, Maijnen CAM, Kranenbarg EK, van de Velde CJK, van Krieken JHM: Circumferential margin involvement is still an important predictor of local recurrence in rectal carcinoma. Not one millimeter but two millimeters is the limit. Am J Surg Pathol 2002;26:350–357.
29 Birbeck KF, Macklin GP, Tiffin NJ, Parsons W, Dixon MF, Mapstone NP, Abbott CR, Scott N, Finan PJ, Johnston D, Quirke P: Rates of circumferential resection margin involvement vary between surgeons and predict outcomes in rectal cancer surgery. Ann Surgery 2002;235:449–457.
30 Adam IJ, Mohamdee MO, Martin IG: Role of circumferential margin involvement in the local recurrence of rectal cancer. Lancet 1994;344:707–11.

31 Wibe A, Rendedal PR, Svensson E, Norstein J, Eide TJ, Myrvold HE, Soreide O: Prognostic significance of the circumferential resection margin following total mesorectal excision for rectal cancer. Br J Surg 2002;89: 327–334.
32 Madoff RD, Sharon L, Dykes, MD: What's new in colon and rectal surgery. J Am Coll Surg 2004;198:91–104.
33 Wibe A, Syse A, Andersen E, Tretli S, Myrvold HE, Soreide O, Norwegian Rectal Cancer Group: Oncological outcomes after total mesorectal excision for cure for cancer lower rectum: anterior vs. abdominoperineal resection. Dis Colon Rectum 2004;47:48–58.
34 Hermanek P, Wittekind C: The pathologist and the residual tumor (R) classification. Pathol Res Pract 1994;190:115–123.
35 Kapiteijn E, Marijnen CA, Nagteggal ID, et al: Preoperative radiotherapy combined with total mesorectal excision for respectable rectal cancer. N Engl J Med 2001;345: 638–646.
36 Oberholzen K, Junginger T, Kreitner KF, Krummenauer F, Simiantonaki N, Trouet S, Thelen M: Local staging of rectal carcinoma and assessment of the circumferential resection margin with high-resolution MRI using an integrated parallel acquisition technique. J Magn Reson Imaging 2005;22:101–108.
37 Mathur P, Smith JJ, Ramsey C, Owen M, Thorpe A, Karim S, Burke C, Ramesh S, Dawson PM: Comparison of CT and MRI in the preoperative staging of rectal adenocarcinoma and prediction of circumferential resection margin involvement by MRI. Colorectal Dis 2003;5:396–401.
38 Beets-Tan RGH, Beets GL: Rectal cancer: review with emphasis on MRI. Radiology 2004;232:335–346.

Review Article

Digestive Diseases

Dig Dis 2007;25:56–66
DOI: 10.1159/000099171

Neoadjuvant Radiochemotherapy for Rectal Cancer

Louiza Vini

Department of Radiotherapy, Athens Medical Center, Athens, Greece

Key Words
Rectal cancer · Radiotherapy · Chemotherapy · Toxicity

Abstract
During the past few decades, significant progress has been achieved in the management of rectal cancer with the introduction of total mesorectal excision. The role of radiotherapy in improving local control and survival has been investigated extensively. Randomized trials of preoperative radiotherapy reported statistically significant lower local recurrence rates with either short regimens (25 Gy in 5 fractions) or conventionally fractionated regimens (45–50 Gy in 25 fractions) and some also showed a survival improvement. Preoperative radiotherapy appears more effective in terms of local control and toxicity compared to postoperative therapy. Several recent studies show that 5-FU-based chemotherapy enhances tumor response to radiotherapy and preoperative chemoradiotherapy is being increasingly used for stage II and III disease.

There are four major goals in the treatment of a patient with rectal cancer: local control, long-term survival, preservation of anal sphincter, bladder and sexual function and finally maintenance or improvement of quality of life. These goals are best achieved through a multimodality approach delivered by a multidisciplinary team. Surgery remains the cornerstone of all therapy and continues to develop towards the ultimate goals of improved local control maintaining good quality of life. In the early series the local recurrence rates after standard surgery were around 30–50%. With extensive surgical training programs and the introduction of total mesorectal excision (TME), several studies in the 1990s reported rates of 8–15% with TME.

Information concerning the depth of tumor penetration through the rectal wall, lymph node involvement and presence of metastatic disease is of crucial importance when planning a curative treatment. Preoperative staging is used to determine the indication for neoadjuvant treatment. Local excision is likely to be curative for most patients with a tumor limited to the submucosa (T1N0M0), but once the tumor invades the muscularis propria (T2), radical resection is recommended. In patients with transmural and/or node-positive disease (T3/T4 and/or N1), preoperative chemoradiotherapy followed by radical resection according to the principles of TME has become widely accepted [1].

KARGER

Fax +41 61 306 12 34
E-Mail karger@karger.ch
www.karger.com

0257–2753/07/0251–0056$23.50/0

Accessible online at:
www.karger.com/ddi

Dr. Louiza Vini, MD, FRCR
Department of Radiotherapy, Athens Medical Center
GR–151 25 Athens (Greece)
Tel. +30 210 615 7317, Fax +30 210 610 0199
E-Mail lvini@iatriko.gr

Table 1. Randomized trials of preoperative radiotherapy in rectal cancer (controlled trials with a surgery-alone group)

Trial	Total dose Gy	Fractions	BED Gy	Local recurrences (%)		Relative reduction, %
				control group	RT group	
Standard surgery						
MRCI	5	1	7.5	118/275 (43)	125/277 (45)	0
	20	10	20.4		128/272 (47)	0
RTOG	5	1	7.5	33/153 (22)	281/148 (19)	12
Dresden	15.5	5	20.3	9/37 (24)	5/40 (13)	49
St. Marks	15	3	22.5	51/210 (24)	31/185 (17)	29
Essen	25	13	24.0	7/71 (10)	4/56 (7)	30
VASAG II	31.5	18	26.8	40/181 (22)	37/180 (21)	0
Bergen	31.5	18	26.8	31/131 (24)	24/138 (17)	29
VASAG I	20–25	10	27.5	32/87 (37)	27/93 (29)	22
North-West	20	4	30.0	58/141 (41)	26/143 (18)	65
Mainz	34.5	15	35.2	21/106 (20)	8/64 (13)	37
Dutch	34.5	15	35.2	18/50 (36)	7/59 (12)	67
EORTC	34.5	15	35.2	49/175 (28)	24/166 (15)	48
MRC2	40	20	36.0	65/140 (46)	50/139 (36)	22
Brazil	40	20	36.0	16/34 (47)	5/34 (15)	68
Stockholm	25	5	37.5	120/425 (28)	61/424 (14)	50
SRCT	25	5	37.5	150/557 (27)	65/553 (12)	60
TME						
Dutch TME	25	5	37.5	72/907 (8)	23/897 (3)	71

Preoperative Radiotherapy

The rationale for preoperative radiotherapy is: for T3 tumors to sterilize tumor deposits outside the mesorectal fascia, to downstage fixed T4 tumors and make a curative procedure possible and for resectable but low rectal cancers (requiring abdominoperineal resection) to downsize enough for sphincter preservation. Preoperative radiotherapy has the theoretical advantage of treating an undisturbed tumor bed which should have a smaller proportion of hypoxic cells and therefore should be more radiosensitive. In addition, radiation fields are usually smaller and acute and long-term toxicity is not severe [2].

Nineteen randomized studies of preoperative radiotherapy have been published so far (table 1). The surgery-alone group, with a few exceptions, has shown local recurrence rates exceeding 20% (on average 28%). Most of these trials showed statistically significant lower local recurrence rates (local recurrence was reduced by 40–50% with preoperative radiotherapy). Radiotherapy was given either with conventional dose and fractionation (20–25 fractions of 1.8–2 Gy to a total dose of 45–50 Gy) or as a short schedule of 5 fractions of 5 Gy each (total dose 25 Gy). Reduction in local failure was seen with both regimens [3]. The two fractionation schedules have not been directly compared and it is not known which is the most effective. The short scheme of preoperative radiotherapy is certainly convenient for the patients without significantly increased acute toxicity. It has a proven efficacy in local tumor control as has most recently been shown by the Dutch trial. A cost utility analysis reported a cost-effectiveness ratio of USD 25,000 per quality-adjusted life-year. However, this scheme does not contribute to downstaging of locally advanced rectal tumors, and it cannot be administered concomitantly with chemotherapy while there is some concern regarding late toxicity.

Three meta-analyses confirmed the significant effect of preoperative radiotherapy on local failure and deaths from rectal cancer. The meta-analysis published in 2001 by the Colorectal Cancer Cooperative Group showed that preoperative radiotherapy at biological doses of >30 Gy reduces the risk of local recurrence by 46%, the 5-year overall mortality by 16% and cancer-related mortality by 29% (table 2). The effect was seen in all stages and both genders. However, the magnitude of benefit on survival is relatively small and criteria are needed to identify patients most likely to benefit from radiotherapy [3].

Table 2. Colorectal cancer collaborative group overview (2001) on randomized trials of preoperative radiotherapy in rectal cancer (meta-analysis of individual patient data)

Aim/study question	Patient population		Results			Conclusion/comments
			%	SE	p	
Surgery alone vs. surgery and preop. or postop. RT, meta-analysis of 22 trials	Trials starting before 1987, 22 of 28 identified trials allowed analyses of individual patient data. 6,360 pts (92% of all) in 14 preop. trials, 2,157 pts (99%) in 8 postop. trials		Reduced overall death rate			Preop. RT (at BED >30 Gy) reduces the risk of local failures and deaths from rectal cancer. The reduction was seen in all stages and both sexes. It increases non-rectal cancer deaths, being technique dependent. The effect on overall survival is limited.
		Preop. BED <20 Gy	5.5	9.4	0.6	
		Preop. 20–30 Gy	0.5	5.3	0.9	
		Preop. >30 Gy	9.8	4.7	0.04	
		Preop. all	5.6	2.9	0.09	
		Postop. all (>35 Gy)	4.6	5.9	0.4	
			Reduced rectal cancer death rate			
		Preop. BED <20 Gy	11.2	11.4	0.3	
		Preop. 20–30 Gy	1.1	6.3	0.9	
		Preop. >30 Gy	21.6	5.1	0.00002	
		Preop. all	12.9	3.7	0.0006	
		Preop. all (>35 Gy)	8.6	6.5	0.2	
			Relative reduction isolated local failure			Preop. RT (at BED 20–30 Gy) slight reduction local failures, no influence on survival. No significant effects are seen using lower preop. doses (BED <20 Gy). Postop. RT (at BED >35 Gy) reduces risk of local failure (less than preop. RT). No influence on survival. M1
		Preop. BED <20 Gy	–20.2	28.8	0.05 adverse	
		Preop. 20–30 Gy	23.7	14.5	0.10	
		Preop. >30 Gy	57.4	6.6	<0.00001	
		Preop. all	46.0	6.0	<0.00001	
		Postop. all (>35 Gy)	36.9	9.7	0.00002	
			Absolute reduction isolated local failures at 5 years			
		Preop. all	22.2–12.5		<0.00001	
		Postop. all	22.9–15.3		<0.0002	
			Increase in non-rectal cancer death rate			
		Preop. BED <20 Gy	–9	16.2	0.8 adverse	
		Preop. 20–30 Gy	–0.8	9.7	0.9 adverse	
		Preop. >30 Gy	–37.2	11.6	0.001 adverse	
		Preop. all	–15.2	6.8	0.02 adverse	
		Postop. all (>35 Gy)	–12.4	14.3	0.1 adverse	

One of the largest studies conducted in the 1980s, the Swedish Rectal Cancer Trial, randomized 1,168 patients with all-stage resectable disease to short-course preoperative radiotherapy (25 Gy in 5 fractions) followed by standard surgery within 1 week of surgery only [4]. In the most recent report with a median follow-up of 13 years, the local recurrence rate was statistically lower following preoperative radiotherapy (9 vs. 26% in the non-irradiated group). The reduction in the local recurrence rate was observed at all tumor locations, although it was not statistically significant for tumors >10 cm from the anal verge. In addition, preoperative radiotherapy resulted in a significant increase in the overall 13-year survival from 30 to 38% and in the cancer-specific survival from 62 to 72%.

In the past decade, it has repeatedly been claimed that surgery was not optimal in the trials that recruited patients in the 1980s. Concentration of rectal cancer surgery to a rectal cancer unit and extensive surgical training programs have resulted in low local recurrence rates only with TME. To investigate the necessity of preoperative radiotherapy with appropriate surgery, the Dutch Colorectal Cancer Group randomized 1,861 patients with resectable rectal cancer to short-course preoperative radiotherapy (25 Gy in 5 fractions in 1 week) immediately followed by TME or TME alone [5]. The study was conducted with the use of standardization and quality control measures to ensure the consistency of surgery, radiotherapy and pathology techniques. With a median follow-up of 2 years, local recurrence was seen in 8.2% following surgery only and 2.4% with the addition of radiotherapy, although overall survival was similar in both groups (82%). The effect was seen for stage II and III tumors located up to 10 cm from the anal verge.

Tumor Response

The effect of radiotherapy on tumor characteristics (reduction in size, necrosis, fibrosis), and consequently on the occurrence of downstaging, depends on treat-

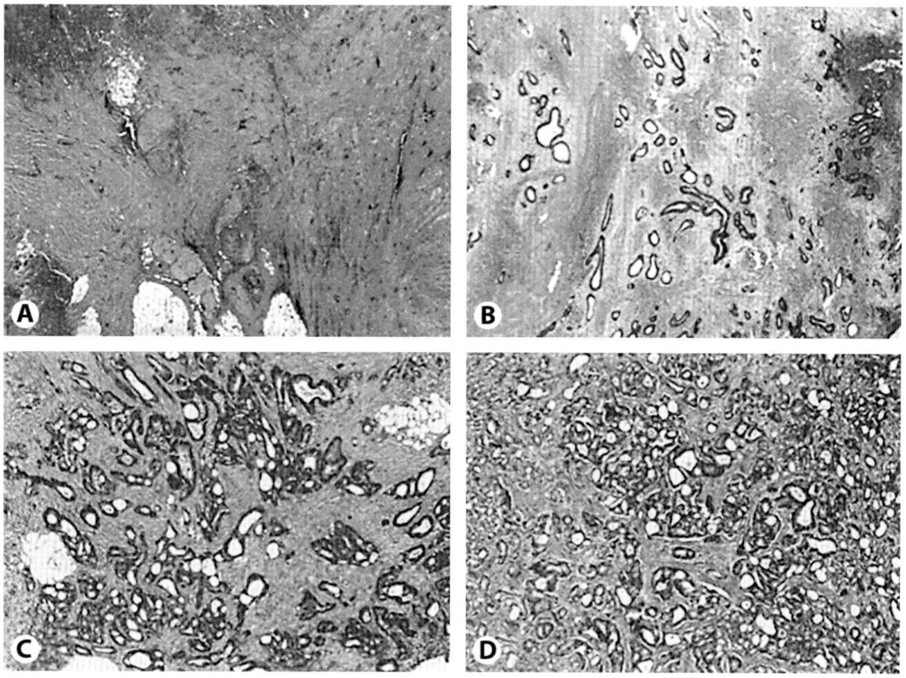

Fig. 1. TRG after preoperative chemoradiotherapy in rectal cancer patients: **A** total regression, no viable tumor cells, only fibrotic mass, TRG 4; **B** dominant fibrosis outgrowing the tumor mass (i.e., >50% tumor regression), TRG 3; **C** dominant tumor mass with obvious fibrosis in 26–50% of the tumor mass, TRG 2; **D** minor regression, fibrosis in only 25% or less of the tumor mass, TRG 1.

ment-related factors as well as tumor-related factors. The total radiation dose, the fraction size, the concomitant administration of chemotherapy and the overall treatment time are associated with tumor response. There is some evidence for a dose-response relationship for rectal cancer. The 2001 Overview indicates that radiotherapy schemes at biological doses >30 Gy are associated with lower recurrence rates improving local disease control by 27% while lower doses have no significant effect on local control [3]. In addition, the Lyon R0-02 trial showed that dose escalation with contact radiotherapy to 85 Gy increased tumor response; mean tumor diameter was decreased from 3.2 to 2.4 cm and the rate of pathologic complete response increased from 2 to 29%. As a result, a sphincter-saving procedure was performed in 79% of patients [6].

In studies in which radiotherapy is delivered as a short scheme of 5 fractions, the overall treatment time is 2 weeks at the most. The interval is too short for the tumor cells to disappear. Analysis of the pathologic tumor characteristics of patients who participated in the Dutch trial showed a small reduction in tumor size, probably due to intratumoral lymphocytic cell death by apoptosis, and the number of recovered lymph nodes but no change in tumor and node classification [7]. Therefore, no downstaging occurs after short-term preoperative radiotherapy. With doses of >40 Gy given with conventional fractionation followed by surgery several weeks later, there is enough time for tumor cells to die resulting in considerable shrinkage. The Lyon R90-01 trial was specifically designed to answer the question of the interval between the end of radiotherapy and surgery and showed a significant increase in tumor response with a long interval of 6 weeks [8].

Assessment of response to radiotherapy by comparing preoperative staging, with endorectal ultrasound, computer tomography or magnetic resonance scans, is likely to overestimate the degree of downstaging. An alternative method is by grading histological changes in the resected specimen. A new system for assessment of tumor response has been recently developed, the tumor regression grading (TRG) scoring with 5 categories, determined by the amount of viable tumor versus fibrosis (fig. 1). TRG was evaluated on surgical specimens of patients treated within the German trial [9]. It was found that complete regression of the primary (TRG 4) was associated with better control of disease in the lymph nodes, sustained local control (100%) and a minor risk to develop distant metastases (DFS 86%). Patients showing an intermediate regression (TRG 2+3) also had an intermediate prognosis (DFS 72%) and poor tumor regression (TRG 0+1) was associated with adverse pathologic features and predicted for an unfavorable outcome (DFS 63%). Although TRG seemed promising in the univariate

Table 3. EORTC 22921 trial: patients' pathological characteristics

Tumor size, mm			
Median	30.0	25.0	p < 0.0001
90% range	10.0–70.0	8.0–110.0	
Tumor stage, patients (%)			
0	25 (5.3)	65 (13.7)	p < 0.001
1	36 (7.6)	49 (10.4)	
2	141 (29.6)	156 (33.0)	
3	233 (48.9)	175 (37.0)	
4	25 (5.3)	18 (3.8)	
Missing	16 (3.4)	10 (2.1)	
Nodes examined			
Mean	9	7	p = 0.046
Range	0.0–45.0	0.0–39	
N stage, n (%)			
N0	288 (60.5)	340 (71.9)	
N1	108 (22.7)	84 (17.8)	
N2	57 (12.0)	34 (7.2)	p < 0.001

analysis, the most important independent prognostic factor for DFS was the pathological T category and the nodal status. In a study from Canada, the post-treatment TNM stage was also a strong prognostic factor for recurrence and survival [10]. By contrast, in a similar study from Padova, tumor response following preoperative chemoradiotherapy was mainly related to the regimen used and only the pretreatment TNM stage was prognostic for the outcome [11].

Adding 5-FU and leucovorin concomitantly with the radiotherapy course significantly decreases tumor size and pTN stage. In most trials of preoperative radiotherapy the complete response rate is around 5–10%, the addition though of chemotherapy resulted in tumor sterilization in 20–30% of patients. Chemotherapy also reduces lymphatic, venous and perineural invasions which have been shown to impact negatively on the outcome while it increases mucin production by the tumors which is considered as a mode of response to therapy [12]. The large EORTC 22921 randomized trial indicates a synergistic effect of chemotherapy on downsizing and downstaging but longer follow-up is needed to assess the impact on local control and survival (table 3).

It seems, therefore, that tumor regression after preoperative chemoradiotherapy is a multifactorial phenomenon. Apart from treatment-related factors, it appears to be associated with smaller, less aggressive disease, and may correspond to the molecular tumor profile regulating tumor response. Apoptosis, apoptosis-related proteins, genes and growth factors may be implicated.

Sphincter-Saving Procedures

Theoretically, the reduction of the tumor bulk induced by preoperative irradiation should improve sphincter preservation in patients with low-lying cancers. This notion seems to be supported by the results of several phase II and two phase III studies [6, 8, 13, 14]. It has also been suggested that the anterior resection rate increases with concurrent chemoradiotherapy. The very recent review of 10 randomized trials involving 4,596 patients showed that tumor shrinkage did not result in a statistically significant higher anterior resection rate (table 4). Subgroups of patients considered to be candidates for abdominoperineal resection before randomization were identified in three trials. A statistically significant higher rate of sphincter-saving procedures was demonstrated in the German trial; however, sphincter preservation was a secondary endpoint [15]. The benefit of sphincter preservation was not confirmed by subgroup analysis in the Lyon R90-01 nor in the Polish study, which were originally designed to address this issue [8, 13].

It should be acknowledged that these trials differed in respect to radiochemotherapy regimens, interval between radiotherapy and surgery, patient populations and the periods of accrual. The distance between the anorectal ring and the lower pole of the tumor certainly lengthens following treatment; however, many surgeons do not perform an anterior resection. One reason might be that they are not convinced by the suggestion of possibility of a shorter surgical distal bowel margin (<1 cm instead of the usually recommended 1–2 cm). In three retrospective studies, there was no association between the length of the distal margin and the risk of local recurrence [16]. By contrast, in many phase II studies, which are single-center studies, the surgeons agreed that the final decision on sphincter preservation has to be based on the tumor status at the time of surgery and not before irradiation and have shown a much higher rate of conservative procedures.

Combined Radiochemotherapy

The rationale for systemic chemotherapy for stage II/III rectal cancer is twofold: 5-FU-based chemotherapy can enhance tumor response to radiotherapy, acting as

Table 4. The AR rates in the randomized trials for respectable rectal adenocarcinoma, in which preoperative irradiation, with or without chemotherapy, resulted in a smaller primary tumor, prior to surgery in the experimental group as compared to the control group

A study name or a name of first author, year of beginning of accrual remarks	Overall quality score[a]	Treatment regimens: experimental group vs. control group	The evidences for tumor shrinkage and higher percentage of CR in an experimental group compared to a control group, respectively, p value	Experimental group no. of patients with ARs/total no. of patients[b] (%)	Control group no. of patients with ARs/total no. of patients[b] (%)	% of treatment effect[c] (95% CI) p value
Trials in which a rate of ARs was the primary endpoint						
Lyon R90-01, 1991	100	The same preoperative irradiation in both groups (39 Gy, 3 Gy/fraction); interval to surgery 6–8 weeks vs. <2 weeks	Clinical PR + CR: 72 vs. 53%, p = 0.007	77/102 (76)	67/99 (68)	8 (–5, +20) 0.27
Polish trial, 1999	100	Preoperative chemoradiation (50.4 Gy, 1.8 Gy/fraction + 2 cycles of 5-Fu, LV, 4–6 weeks interval to surgery vs. preoperative 5 × 5 Gy, immediate surgery	Mean dimension of tumors along bowel axis: 26 vs. 45 mm, p < 0.001; clinical CR: 13 vs. 3%, p < 0.001	91/157 (58)	94/154 (61)	–3 (–14, +8) 0.64
Trials in which a rate of ARs was a secondary endpoint						
CAO/ARO/AIO 94, 1994 Analysis according to actual treatment given	80	Preoperative chemoradiation (50.4 Gy, 1.8 Gy/fraction + 2 cycles of 5-Fu, LV, up to 8 weeks interval to surgery vs. postoperative chemoradiation	Downstaging (p < 0.001)	286/415 (69)	273/384 (71)	–2 (–9, +4) 0.54
NSABP R-03, 1993 40% (45/113) of patients were excluded from analysis	50	1 cycle of 5-Fu, LV + preoperative chemoradiation (50.4 Gy, 1.8 Gy/fraction + 2 cycles of 5-Fu, LV, up to 8 weeks interval to surgery) vs. postoperative chemoradiation	Downstaging: pathological CR + stage I: 33 vs. 16%, p value not given	15/31 (48)	11/37 (30)	+19 (–4, +42) 0.14
Trials in which a rate of ARs was not an endpoint						
MRC 1, 1975 Three-arm study; in single fraction preoperative group no downsizing was seen and therefore this group was combined with surgery-only group	80	Preoperative irradiation 20 Gy, 2 Gy/fraction, interval to surgery <1 week vs. surgery alone or single fraction 5 Gy within 1 week before surgery	Tumor size >4 cm: 46% for multiple fraction group vs. 61% for surgery alone + single fraction group, p = 0.004	57/272 (21)	133/548 (24)	–3 (–9, +3) 0.29
Horn, 1976	33	Preoperative irradiation 31.5 Gy, 1.75 Gy/fraction, interval to surgery 2–3 weeks vs. surgery alone	Median tumor diameter: 32 vs. 43 mm, p < 0.05	50/157 (32)	51/149 (34)	–2 (–13, +8) 0.72
Reis Neto, 1978	0	Preoperative irradiation 40 Gy, 2 Gy/fraction, interval to surgery 1 week vs. surgery alone	After radiotherapy 76% of patients had the tumor mass reduction more than 70% of its initial size	18/34 (53)	22/34 (65)	–12 (–35, +12) 0.27
MRC 2, 1981	100	Preoperative irradiation 40 Gy, 2 Gy/fraction, interval to surgery at least 4 weeks vs. surgery alone	Tumor size >4 cm: 32 vs. 64%, p < 0.001	46/139 (33)	52/140 (37)	–4 (–15, +7) 0.53
EORTC 22921, 1993	100	Preoperative chemoradiation (2 cycles of 5-Fu, LV) vs. preoperative irradiation alone; 45 Gy, 1.8 Gy/fraction and interval to surgery 3–10 weeks in both groups	Smaller tumors after chemoradiation, p < 0.001	263/506 (52)	249/505 (49)	+3 (–4, +9) 0.41
FFCD 9203, 1993	Abstract, assessment is not possible	Preoperative chemoradiation (2 cycles of 5-Fu, LV) vs. preoperative irradiation alone; 45 Gy, 1.8 Gy/fraction and interval to surgery 3–10 weeks in both groups	Clinical CR: 5.7 vs. 2.6%, NS pathological CR: 11.7 vs. 3.7%, p < 0.0001	184/370 (50)	182/363 (50)	0 (–8, +7) 0.94

AR = Anterior resection; CR = complete response; PR = partial response; NS = non-significant.
[a] In order to assessing the quality of trials, the scores attached to each individual item of domains of concealment of treatment allocation and handling of with drawals were summed to produce an overall quality score as the percentage of the maximum score theoretically achievable. [b] Patients who underwent local excision were excluded. Total number of these patients was: experimental arm 3 (0.1%), control arm 8 (0.3%). The number of patients treated with Hartmann's procedures was included in numerators. Total number of these patients was: experimental arm 17 (0.8%), control arm 32 (1.3%). [c] Treatment effect equals: anterior resection rate in experimental arm minus anterior resection rate in control arm; '+' denotes treatment effect better in experimental group, '–' worse in experimental group.

radiosensitizer, and adjuvant systemic chemotherapy for node-positive or high-risk patients can reduce distant relapse rates and improve survival. The proper sequence and combination of treatment modalities is controversial. Over the past two decades, randomized trials in North America have shown the efficacy of postoperative radiotherapy and chemotherapy.

The Gastrointestinal Tumor Study Group trial was the first to show local recurrence, disease-free and overall survival benefit with combination of chemotherapy and radiotherapy in high-risk stage II/III rectal cancers [17]. These results were further supported by the Mayo Clinic Study. The National Cancer Institute Consensus Conference in 1990 concluded that combined modality therapy should be administered to patients with stage II/III rectal cancer [18]. However, these results were not seen in other trials. Of note, the two recent studies from the NSABP R02 and a study from Italy showed decreased local failure rates but no effect on survival. One interesting study showed that protracted venous infusion of 5-FU during radiotherapy improved survival compared to intermittent bolus injections, this could be related to prolonged tumor cell exposure to drug or to higher total doses of 5-FU [19]. Some other phase II and III studies showed no benefit from combination chemotherapy compared to 5-FU alone [20].

In the 1990s there were some indications that preoperative was more effective than postoperative radiotherapy in terms of local control. The study by Frykholm et al. [21] reported lower local failure rate after preoperative compared to postoperative radiotherapy (13 and 22%, respectively); however, there was no difference in survival between the two groups. Two recent studies, INT 0145 and NSABP 03, closed early because of insufficient accrual, but the German Rectal Cancer Group Trial comparing preoperative to postoperative combined chemoradiotherapy was published in 2004 with a median follow-up of 45 months [15]. A 5-year cumulative incidence of local failure of 6% was seen in the preoperative RT arm compared to 13% in the postoperative RT arm, a statistically significant difference, while overall 5-year survival was 76 and 74%, respectively. Toxicity was worse in the postoperative arm with 40% grade 3–4 toxic events compared to 27%.

At the beginning of the 1990s, it became clear that preoperative chemoradiotherapy was a relevant issue for clinical research. The EORTC radiotherapy group demonstrated that a 5-FU dose of 350 mg/m^2/day could be safely administered in combination with a leucovorin dose of 20 mg/m^2/day during the first and fifth week of

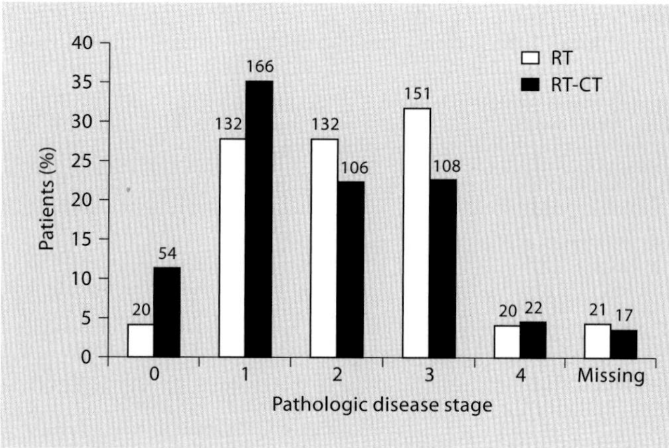

Fig. 2. EORTC 22921 trial. Pathologic disease stage.

radiotherapy to a total dose of 45 Gy. Later the EORTC conducted the four-arm trial 22921 to examine the value of preoperative radiochemotherapy versus preoperative radiotherapy alone and the value of additional postoperative chemotherapy versus none with respect to overall survival and progression-free survival [12]. Preliminary analysis published in 2005 showed that the addition of 5-FU and LV chemotherapy reduced tumor size and pathological stage with slightly increased acute toxicity (fig. 2). The compliance with the radiotherapy protocol and the feasibility of surgery did not decrease. Longer follow-up is needed to assess the true impact on local control and survival. The trial conducted by the Fédération Francophone de Cancérologie Digestive compared preoperative chemoradiotherapy with 5-FU and folinic acid versus radiotherapy and reported lower local recurrence rate with combined treatment without any survival benefit [22]. Interestingly, in all studies, no impact was seen on distant metastases with preoperative chemotherapy. Two possible explanations for this observation were that the chemotherapeutic agents used were administered at doses adequate for radiosensitizing local effect but not adequate to have a systemic effect, and that 5-FU and leucovorin were suboptimal chemotherapy agents.

Several agents are currently being evaluated for their role in an integrated treatment program. These include oral fluoropyrimidines such as Xeloda, irinotecan (CPT-11), oxaliplatin and cetuximab, which is a monoclonal antibody against the epidermal growth factor receptor. Xeloda mimics continuous infusion of 5-FU. The enzyme thymidine phosphorylase is essential for the activation of Xeloda. This is more active in tumor than in normal tissue while radiotherapy upregulates TP in tumor and re-

Table 5. Radiotherapy alone combined with radiotherapy plus chemotherapy in non-resectable rectal cancer

Author/year/design	Aim/study question	Patient population	Results	Conclusion/comments
Moertel, 1969 C	A: RT 35–40 Gy + placebo B: RT 35–40 Gy + 5-FU	A: 33 pts B: 32 pts	Mean survival, months A: 17 B: 25, $p < 0.05$ 3-year survival A: 9% B: 19%, n.s.	Colon and rectum together (the study also included patients with gastric and pancreatic cancer). This study was interpreted early to show that RTCHT (3 days of 5-FU) was superior to RT alone. C3
Rominger, 1985 C	A: RT 45–51 Gy + boost B: RT 45–51 Gy + 5-FU maintenance CHT	129/147 evaluable A: 65 pts B: 64 pts	2-year survival A: 36% B: 44%, n.s. No difference in failure pattern More complications in B	No difference between RTCHT and RT, increased risk of complications C3
Overgaard, 1993 C	A: RT 50 Gy + boost B: RT 50 Gy + weekly 5-FU	A: 29 pts B: 30 pts	3-year survival A: 7% B: 16%, n.s. Acute toxicity A: 13% B: 33%, $p = 0.07$	Significant palliation in 73%, no difference between groups, except for more toxicity with RTCHT.
Frykholm, 2001 C	A: 46 Gy RT B: 40 Gy RT split course + methotrexate + 5-FU + leucovorin	A: 36 pts B: 34 pts	LFS at 5 years A: 38% B: 66%, $p = 0.03$ OS at 5 years A: 18% B: 29%, $p = 0.3$	Gives some support to the view that RTCHT is superior to RT, but did not have the same RT schedule in the two arms. C3

sults in more 5-FU in tumor cells. Studies indicate that Xeloda has an additive activity in combination with radiotherapy while it simplifies chemoradiation and is highly appealing to patients. There are currently several ongoing phase II and III studies in the neoadjuvant setting. Combinations with oxaliplatin and irinotecan are also being investigated and may further improve local and systemic control. These agents have improved overall survival in patients with metastatic colorectal cancer and disease-free survival for patients with completely resected stage II and III colon cancer, while oxaliplatin in addition has a radiosensitizing effect.

Many different concurrent chemoradiotherapy regimens have been evaluated in phase I/II studies during the past 5 years. In the Lyon R0-04 trial, two cycles of oxaliplatin and continuous infusion 5-FU during the first and the fifth week of the radiotherapy course (50 Gy in 5 weeks) resulted in objective clinical response in 75% with pathologic complete response in 15% and sphincter-saving surgery was possible in 65% of the patients [23]. A phase I/II study by the Cancer and Leukemia Group B showed that the addition of weekly oxaliplatin 60 mg/m^2 to continuous infusion of 5-FU 200 mg/m^2 during the radiotherapy showed pathologic complete response in 26% of patients with T3/T4 tumors. Toxicity, grade 3 and 4 diarrhea, was increased, but most patients completed therapy as planned [24]. In another study from the Royal Marsden Hospital, patients with locally advanced rectal tumors received 12 weeks of neoadjuvant oxaliplatin/capecitabine chemotherapy followed by concomitant capecitabine and radiotherapy. TME was performed 6 weeks later and postoperatively 12 more weeks of capecitabine were given. Pathologic complete response was documented in 24% and in an additional 48% of patients only microscopic tumor foci were found on surgical specimens. Distant metastases were seen only in 10% of the patients, although the follow-up was relatively short. Toxicity, though, was not negligible with four toxic deaths as a result of pulmonary embolism and ischemic heart disease [25]. In view of this promising activity, two randomized trials (the NSABP 04 and a multicenter study by the MRC UK) have already been initiated and their results will be very helpful.

Management of Fixed Unresectable Tumors

For locally advanced non-resectable rectal cancers, radiotherapy or combined radiotherapy and chemotherapy achieve marked tumor regression in a significant proportion and facilitates resection. Several trials have reported that preoperative radiotherapy or radiochemotherapy results in radical resection in about 40–70% of patients and that 20–30% will become long-term survivors. Four trials have randomly compared radiotherapy alone with 5-FU chemotherapy concurrent with radiotherapy (table 5). These trials are small and do not provide supportive evidence that radiochemotherapy is superior to radiotherapy alone. However, patient selection may be a very important issue for treatment results. Ferrigno et al. [26] treated 101 patients with fixed or semifixed tumors with radiotherapy, 45 Gy to the whole pelvis and 50.4 Gy to the primary, and concomitant weekly chemotherapy with 5-FU and leucovorin. A complete response was seen in 8% and radical tumor removal with negative margins was achieved in 82% of patients. The actuarial 5-year local control was 76% and distant metastasis was the predominant pattern of failure supporting the need for new chemotherapy agents. Pelvic nodal involvement and incomplete excision were the main adverse prognostic factors. For fixed tumors, high-dose rate intraoperative radiotherapy in combination with preoperative external beam radiotherapy and chemotherapy has also been investigated with some very promising early results. Addition of intraoperative therapy for patients with narrow or microscopic incomplete resection seems to overrule the unfavorable prognostic histological finding. A study from The Netherlands reported 5-year local control of 58% and overall survival of 38% for patients with R1/R2 resections [27].

Toxicity

Complications of pelvic radiotherapy are a function of the volume treated, the overall treatment time, fraction size, total dose, radiation energy and technique. Large field sizes, short overall treatment time, large fraction sizes (>2 Gy), low-energy radiation, the use of a two-field technique and the lack of computerized dosimetry all contribute to an increased incidence of radiation complications [2]. Other patient-related risk factors such as pelvic inflammatory disease, diabetes, hypertension, obesity, previous surgery and concurrent chemotherapy also increase the incidence and severity of complications. Willett et al. [28] reported a series of 28 patients with inflammatory bowel disease (18 with ulcerative colitis and 10 with Crohn's disease) treated with pelvic radiotherapy to 40 Gy or more for colorectal cancer. Severe acute toxicity was seen in 46% which caused 22% of patients to stop treatment. Acute toxicity was similar in ulcerative colitis and Crohn's disease; however, late toxicity was limited to patients with ulcerative colitis. For these patients specialized radiation techniques must be used in an effort to reduce total dose or exclude the small and large bowel from the radiation field.

The most frequent complications which occur in almost all patients include effects on the small bowel (diarrhea, cramping), the large bowel (proctitis, tenesmus, bloody or mucus discharge), the bladder (frequency, dysuria) and hematological toxicity (thrombocytopenia, leukopenia). The mechanism is primarily the depletion of actively dividing cells. In the small bowel, loss of mucosal cells results in malabsorption of fat, carbohydrate, protein and bile salts. These symptoms are transient and resolve within a few weeks after the end of radiotherapy. Concurrent chemotherapy increases gastrointestinal and hematological toxicity; acute grade 3+ toxicity occurred in 22% of patients in the chemoradiotherapy arm and in 4% in the radiotherapy only arm in the INT 0114 trial of postoperative combined modality treatment. The addition of chemotherapy increases acute toxicity more in the postoperative setting compared to preoperative. The German Rectal Cancer Group Trial reported 40% grade 3–4 toxic events in the postoperative group and 23% in the preoperative group [15].

Long-term complications occur less frequently about 6–18 months after completion of radiation. Injury to the vascular and supporting stromal tissues of the bowel is the presumed pathophysiology. The most common complications are due to small bowel damage and include enteritis, proctitis, adhesions and small bowel obstruction requiring surgical intervention. In most series the incidence of mild to moderate late complications range from 8 to 15% and is directly proportional to the volume of small bowel in the radiation field. The effect of radiotherapy on sphincter function has not been properly assessed. However, in a recent prospective study preoperative radiotherapy given with conventional dose and technique had a minimal effect on sphincter function [29]. Patients though who received 25 Gy in 5 fractions in the Swedish trial had a significant increase in bowel frequency, incontinence, urgency and emptying difficulty and this impaired patients' social life 30% of the time compared with 10% with surgery alone [30]. Pelvic radiotherapy can also have an adverse effect on sexual function especially if given as a short course. Irradiated males who participated in the Swedish trials had more ejaculation disorders than non-irradiated patients and erectile functioning deteriorated over time [31]. Finally, in the same study, an increased risk for second cancers in the irradiated group was seen in organs within or adjacent to the irradiated volume (relative risk 2.04) but not outside.

Improvements in Radiotherapy

In the past two decades, advances in diagnostic imaging, computer technology and accelerator design have resulted in new radiotherapy techniques such as the three-dimensional conformal technique (3D conformal RT) and the IMRT. These techniques include several aspects: appropriate patient immobilization, simulation using a CT simulator, three-dimensional conformal planning using multiple fields, treatment delivery with a high-energy linear accelerator, use of multileaf collimator to conform the treatment volume to the shape of the target and electronic portal imaging to ensure accurate daily setup. As a result, a homogenous dose distribution is maintained throughout the target volume while minimizing the dose to surrounding normal structures. In a report from the Photon Treatment Planning Collaborative Group, it was found that the most important contribution of the three-dimensional treatment planning in rectal cancer was the ability to localize the target volume and normal tissues at all levels [32]. In addition, a decrease in the volume of normal tissues in the radiation fields was also seen. Attempts are being made to selectively subtract the anal sphincter from the high-dose field in order to improve functioning outcome in patients with mid-rectal tumors scheduled for a low anterior resection [33]. Only lately, the IMRT technique with a five-field customized segmented plan has significantly reduced the volume of small and large bowel irradiated to high dose, which could potentially lead to less bowel toxicity [34].

Conclusions

To conclude:

- Significant progress has been achieved in the treatment of rectal cancer over the past 20 years. Combined modality therapy with the integration of optimal surgery, radiotherapy and chemotherapy has resulted in a significant reduction in local recurrence rates and also an improved survival.
- Optimizing outcome after treatment includes minimizing both the recurrence rate and the number of cancer-related deaths, as well as maximizing patients' quality of life. Yet, even as we await future trials to refine our treatment strategies, we must ensure best practices for patients with rectal cancer today.
- Preoperative staging is important and imaging by endorectal ultrasound or magnetic resonance should be routine.
- Surgery for rectal cancer should be performed by surgeons with training in the technique of TEM and adequate experience.
- Finally, pelvic radiotherapy should be planned and delivered by optimal technique and both radiotherapy and surgery need to be coordinated with evolving chemotherapy regimens.

References

1 Balch GC, De Meo A, Guiillem JG: Modern management of rectal cancer: a 2006 update. World J Gastroenterol 2006;28:3186–3195.

2 Gerard JP: Radiotherapy in the conservative management of rectal cancer. Evidence-based medicine and opinion. Radiother Oncol 2005;74:227–233.

3 Colorectal Cancer Collaborative Group: Adjuvant radiotherapy for rectal cancer a systemic overview of 8,507 patients from 22 randomised trials. Lancet 2001;358:1291–1304.

4 Folkesson J, Birgisson H, Palhman L, et al: Swedish Rectal Cancer Trial: long-lasting benefits from radiotherapy on survival and local recurrence rate. Clin Oncol 2005;23:5644–5650.

5 Kapiteijin E, Marijnen CM, Nagtegaal ID, et al: Preoperative radiotherapy combined with total mesorectal excision for resectable rectal cancer. N Engl J Med 2001;345:638–646.

6 Gerard JP, Chapet O, Nemoz C, et al: Improved sphincter preservation in low rectal cancer with high-dose preoperative radiotherapy: the Lyon R0-02 trial. J Clin Oncol 2004;22:2404–2409.

7 Marijnen CA, Nagtegaal E, Kelin-Kranenbarg E, et al: No downstaging after short-term preoperative radiotherapy in rectal cancer patients. J Clin Oncol 2001;19:1976–1984.

8 Francois Y, Nemoz CJ, Baulieux J, et al: Influence of the interval between preoperative radiation therapy and surgery on downstaging and on the rate of sphincter-saving surgery for rectal cancer: the Lyon R90-01 randomised trial. J Clin Oncol 1999;17:2396–2402.

9 Rodel C, Marus P, Papadopoulos T, et al: Prognostic significance of tumour regression after preoperative chemoradiotherapy for rectal cancer. J Clin Oncol 2005;23:8688–8696.
10 Chan AK, Wong A, Jenken D, et al: Posttreatment TNM staging is a prognostic indicator of survival and recurrence in tethered or fixed rectal carcinoma after preoperative chemotherapy and radiotherapy. Int J Radiat Oncol Biol Phys 2005;1:665–677.
11 Pucciarelli S, Toppan P, Frisso ML, et al: Complete pathologic response following preoperative chemoradiotherapy for middle to lower rectal cancer is not a prognostic indicator for a better outcome. Dis Colon Rectum 2004;47:1798–1807.
12 Bosset JF, Calais G, Mineur L, et al: Enhanced tumouricidal effect of chemotherapy with preoperative radiotherapy for rectal cancer. Preliminary results of EORTC 22921. J Clin Oncol 2005;23:5620–5627.
13 Bujko K, Nowacki MP, Nasierowska-Guttmejer A, et al: Sphincter preservation following preoperative radiotherapy for rectal cancer: report of a randomised trial comparing short-term radiotherapy vs. conventionally fractionated radiochemotherapy. Radiother Oncol 2004;72:15–24.
14 Bujko K, Kepka L, Michalski W, Nowacki MP: Does rectal radiotherapy shrinkage induced by preoperative radiochemotherapy increase the likelihood of anterior resection? A systematic review of randomised trials. Radiother Oncol 2006;80:4–12.
15 Sauer R, Becker H, Hohenberger W, et al: Preoperative versus postoperative chemoradiotherapy for rectal cancer. N Engl J Med 2004;351:1731–1740.
16 Moore HG, Riedel E, Minsky BD, et al: Adequacy of 1 cm distal margin after restorative rectal cancer resection with sharp mesorectal excision and preoperative combined modality therapy. Ann Surg Oncol 2003;10: 80–85.
17 Gastrointestinal Tumour Study Group: Prolongation of the disease-free survival in surgically treated rectal carcinoma. N Engl J Med 1985;312:1465–1472.
18 Guillem JG, Chessin DB, Cohen AM, et al: Long-term oncologic outcome following preoperative combined modality therapy and total mesorectal excision of locally advanced rectal cancer. Ann Surg 2005;241: 829–838.
19 O'Connell MJ, Martenson JA, Wieand HS, et al: Improving adjuvant therapy for rectal cancer by combining protracted infusion fluorouracil with radiation therapy after curative surgery. N Engl J Med 1994:331:502–507.
20 Crane CH, Skibber J, Birnbaum E, et al: The addition of continuous infusion 5-FU to preoperative radiation therapy increases tumour response leading to increased sphincter preservation in locally advanced rectal cancer. Int J Radiat Oncol Biol Phys 2003;57: 84–89.
21 Frykholm GJ, Glimelius B, Palman L: Combined chemo- and radiotherapy vs. radiotherapy alone in the treatment of primary nonresectable adenocarcinoma of the rectum. Int J Radiat Oncol Biol Phys 2001;50: 427–434.
22 Gerard JP, Bonnetain F, Conroy T, et al: Preoperative radiotherapy +/– 5-FU/folinic acid in T3 rectal cancers. Results of the FFCD 9203 randomised trial. J Clin Oncol 2005; 23(suppl):247, abstr 3504.
23 Gerard JP, Chapet O, Nemoz C, et al: Preoperative concurrent chemoradiotherapy in locally advanced rectal cancer with high-dose radiation and oxaliplatin-containing regimen: the Lyon R0-04 phase II trial. J Clin Oncol. 2003;21:1119–1124.
24 Ryan D, Niedzwicki D, Hollis D, et al: A phase I/II study of preoperative oxaliplatin, fluorouracil and external beam radiation therapy in patients with locally advanced rectal cancer: Cancer and Leukemia Group B 89901. J Clin Oncol 2006;24:1–5.
25 Chau J, Brown G, Cunningham D, et al: Neoadjuvant capecitabine and oxaliplatin followed by synchronous chemoradiation and total mesorectal excision in magnetic resonance imaging poor-risk rectal cancer. J Clin Oncol 2006;24:668–674.
26 Ferrigno R, Novaes PE, Silva ML, et al: Neoadjuvant radiochemotherapy in the treatment of fixed and semifixed rectal tumours. Analysis of results and prognostic factors. Radiat Oncol 2006;1:5.
27 Ferenschild FT, Vermaas M, Nuyttens JJ, et al: Value of intraoperative radiotherapy in locally advanced rectal cancer. Dis Colon Rectum 2006;49:1257–1265
28 Willett CG, Ooi CJ, Zeitman AL, et al: Acute and late toxicity of patients with inflammatory bowel disease undergoing irradiation for abdominal and pelvic malignancies. Int J Radiat Oncol Biol Phys 2000;46:995–998.
29 Birnbaum EH, Dreznik Z, Myerson RJ, et al: Early effects of external beam radiation on anal sphincter: a study using anal manometry and transrectal ultrasound. Dis Colon Rectum 1992;35:757–761.
30 Marijnen CA, van de Velde CP, Putter H, et al: Impact of short-term preoperative radiotherapy on health-related quality of life and sexual functioning in primary rectal cancer: report of a multicenter randomised trial. J Clin Oncol 2005;23:1847–1858.
31 Fisher SE, Daniels IR: Quality of life and sexual function following surgery for rectal cancer. Colorectal Dis 2006;8:40–42.
32 Roels S, Duthoy W, Haustermans K, et al: Definition and delineation of the clinical target volume for rectal cancer. Int J Radiat Oncol Biol Phys 2006,65:1129–1142.
33 Gervaz P, Lavertu S, Kazemba B, et al: Sphincter-preserving radiation therapy for rectal cancer: a simulation study using three-dimensional computerized technology. Colorectal Dis 2006;5:570–574.
34 Guerrero-Urbano MT, Henrys AJ, Adams EJ, et al: Intensity modulated radiotherapy in patients with locally advanced rectal cancer reduces volume of bowel treated to high dose levels. Int J Radiat Oncol Biol Phys 2006;65: 907–916.

Review Article

Digestive Diseases

Dig Dis 2007;25:67–75
DOI: 10.1159/000099172

Adjuvant Chemotherapy for Colon Cancer: Evidence on Improvement in Survival

E. Samantas[a] C. Dervenis[b] S.K. Rigatos[a]

[a]Third Oncology Department, 'Agii Anargiri' Cancer Hospital, and [b]First Department of Surgery, 'Agia Olga' Hospital, Athens, Greece

Key Words
Colon cancer · Adjuvant chemotherapy · Fluoropyrimidines

Abstract
Clear progress has been made in the adjuvant treatment of colon cancer. Until very recently, the absolute benefit for survival obtained with the administration of 6 months' FU/LV compared with control was about 6%. Fluoropyrimidines have been shown to be at least as active and can replace intravenous FU/LV in stage III colon cancer. Based on the results of the MOSAIC and NSABP C-07 trials, the addition of oxaliplatin to FU/LV improves disease-free survival and FOLFOX for 6 months can be recommended as adjuvant treatment for patients with stage III colon cancer. The benefit of adjuvant chemotherapy in stage II disease is limited and it should be proposed in patients with high-risk features. Adjuvant treatment of colon cancer improving and the use of genetic/molecular markers with the new targeted therapies may further improve survival.

Introduction

Colorectal cancer (CRC) accounts for 10–15% of all cancers and is the second leading cause of cancer-related death in Western countries [1]. Surgery is the primary treatment modality with curative intent in locoregionally advanced colon cancer. However, 40–50% of the operated patients will relapse and require further treatment. [2]. Every year, CRC is responsible for an estimated 400,000 deaths worldwide. Clinical failure following rejection of colon cancer is predominantly a result of previously undetected residual or metastatic disease. Colon cancer is not uniformly fatal and there are large differences in survival depending on the stage of disease. The pathologic stage is currently the most important determinant of prognosis. The classification systems described by the Dukes no longer fulfill the requirements of modern tumor staging. It does not take into account distant metastases, the number of lymph modes involved or cancers limited to the submucosa. The TNM classification system is currently recommended. The updated sixth edition of the American Joint Committee on Cancer stratifies colon cancer stages II and III by use of T stage and N stage [3].

Adjuvant chemotherapy given after surgery was developed to reduce the risk of disease recurrence, either as local or distant metastases, in patients with stage II/III disease. Relapse of disease occurs in the majority of patients within the first 3 years, with the relapse rate reaching a peak in the second year [4]. The traditional endpoint of adjuvant chemotherapy studies for colon cancer has been 5-year overall survival (OS). A recent analysis of pooled data by Sargent et al. [5] from nearly 13,000 patients with stage III colon cancer found that 3-year disease-free survival (DFS) highly correlated with 5-year

KARGER
Fax +41 61 306 12 34
E-Mail karger@karger.ch
www.karger.com

0257–2753/07/0251–0067$23.50/0

Accessible online at:
www.karger.com/ddi

Dr. E. Samantas
3rd Oncology Department, 'Agii Anargiri' Cancer Hospital
Hassias Av. 9th Station
GR–131 22 Athens (Greece)
Tel./Fax +30 210 238 8798, E-Mail hecogaga@otenet.gr

Table 1. Chemotherapy regimens and dosing in adjuvant colon cancer

Regimen	Drugs and dosage	Frequency	
5-FU/LV-based			
Mayo Clinic	5-FU 425 mg/m^2	Days 1–5	q28 days
	LV 20 mg/m^2	Days 1–5	
Roswell Park	5-FU 500 mg/m^2	Days 1, 8, 15, 22, 29, 36	q8 weeks
	LV 500 mg/m^2	Days 1, 8, 15, 22, 29, 36	
LV5FU2	LV 200 mg/m^2	Days 1, 2	q14 days
	5-FU 400 mg/m^2 bolus	Days 1, 2	
	5-FU 600 mg/m^2 CI 22 h	Days 1, 2	
AIO	LV 500 mg/m^2	Days 1, 8, 15, 22, 29, 36	q8 weeks
	5-FU 2,000 mg/m^2 CI 24 h	Days 1, 8, 15, 22, 29, 36	
Oxaliplatin-based			
FOLFOX 4	OX 85 mg/m^2	Day 1	
	LV 200 mg/m^2	Days 1, 2	q14 days
	5-FU 400 mg/m^2 bolus	Days 1, 2	
	5-FU 600 mg/m^2 CI 22 h	Days 1, 2	
m FOLFOX6	OX 85 mg/m^2	Day 1	
	LV 200 mg/m^2	Days 1	q14 days
	5-FU 400 mg/m^2 bolus	Days 1	
	5-FU 2,400 mg/m^2 CI 46 h	Days 1–2	
FLOX	OX 85 mg/m^2	Days 1, 15, 29	
	LV 500 mg/m^2	Days 1, 8, 15, 22, 29, 36	q8 weeks
	5-FU 500 mg/m^2	Days 1, 8, 15, 22, 29, 36	
XELOX	OX 130 mg/m^2	Day 1	
	CAPE 1,000 mg/m^2 orally BID	Day 1–14	q3 weeks
Irinotecan-based			
IFL	IRI 125 mg/m^2	Days 1, 8, 15, 22	
	LV 20 mg/m^2	Days 1, 8, 15, 22	q6 weeks
	5-FU 500 mg/m^2	Days 1, 8, 15, 22	
FOLFIRI	IRI 180 mg/m^2	Day 1	
	LV 500 mg/m^2	Days 1	q14 days
	5-FU 400 mg/m^2 bolus	Days 1	
	5-FU 2.4–3 g/m^2 CI 46 h	Days 1–2	
IF	IRI 180 mg/m^2	Day 1	
	LV 200 mg/m^2	Days 1, 2	q14 days
	5-FU 400 mg/m^2 bolus	Days 1, 2	
	5-FU 600 mg/m^2 CI 22 h	Days 1, 2	

5-FU = 5-Fluorouracil; BID = twice daily; CAPE = capecitabine; CI = continuous infusion; IRI = irinotecan; LV = leucovorin; OX = oxaliplatin.

OS, suggesting that 3-year DFS is an appropriate primary endpoint for adjuvant chemotherapy studies. Thus, the earlier evidence of clinical and statistical benefit from chemotherapy for colon cancer may lead to earlier translation of clinical trial results into practice. In the 1980s, adjuvant 5-fluorouracil (5-FU)-based chemotherapy was proven to decrease the risk of recurrence from CRC versus observation [6–14]. Since then, many large, well-designed, randomized controlled trials have demonstrated that 5-FU modulation with leucovorin (FU/LV) offers better DFS and OS than other 5-FU modulations [15–20]; that high-dose LV is equally effective with low-dose LV; that the two most commonly administered regimens of bolus 5-FU/LV, Mayo Clinic regimen and weekly Roswell-Park regimen, have similar efficacy [19]; that there is no additional benefit to prolong treatment from 6 to 12 months [21], and that infusional regimens have similar efficacy to bolus regimens but are associated with fewer, severe toxicities [22–24] (table 1). Overall, 5-FU-based adjuvant therapies reduce the risk of recurrence by 30% and the risk of death by 26% over observation [25]. Despite this substantial reduction,

Table 2. Oral fluoropyrimidines in the adjuvant treatment of patients with colon cancer

Trial	Stage	Patients	3/5 years	DFS		3/5 years	RFS		3/5 years	Survival	
				HR	p		HR	p		HR	p
X-Act[a]	III	1,987									
FU/FA			60.6[a]	0.87	0.05	61.9[a]	0.86	0.04	77.6[a]	0.84	0.07
Capecitabine			64.2[a]	(0.75–1.00)		65.5[a]	(0.74–0.99)		81.3[a]	(0.69–1.01)	
NSABP C-06	II/III	1,608									
FU/FA			68.3[b]		0.79	76.4[b]		0.52	78.7[b]		0.88
UFT/FA			66.9[b]			74.5[b]			78.7[b]		

HR = Hazard ratio; FU = fluorouracil; FA = folinic acid; NSABP = National Surgical Adjuvant Breast and Bowel Project; UFT = uracil florafur; DFS = disease-free survival; RFS = relapse-free survival.

[a] 3 years; [b] 5 years.

many patients relapse and succumb from the disease each year, justifying the continuing effort to improve outcomes.

New Drugs

Oral Fluoropyrimidines

Several studies have investigated the activity of oral fluoropyrimidines in the adjuvant treatment of colon cancer. The X-Act study randomly assigned 1,987 patients with resected stage III colon cancer to receive either capecitabine 2,500 mg/m^2 daily, days 1–14 every 21 days or bolus FU/LV (Mayo Clinic regimen) for 6 months [26]. DFS at 3 years was at least equivalent to that in the 5-FU/LV group. Capecitabine improved relapse-free survival and was associated with significantly fewer adverse events than 5-FU/LV. The 3-year survival was 81.3% for capecitabine compared with 77.6% for 5-FU/LV ($p = 0.07$) (table 2).

The NSABP C-06 trial compared intravenous administration of FU/LV in Roswell Park regimen for three cycles with UFT/LV (UFT 300 mg/m^2) daily and LV 90 mg daily, days 1–28, every 35 days for five cycles in 1,608 patients with stage II and III colon cancer [27]. No difference has been observed between the two treatment arms concerning 5-year DFS (66.9 vs. 68.3%) or 5-year OS (78.7 vs. 78.7%). Both regimens had similar toxicity profiles (table 2).

In a meta-analysis of three randomized Japanese studies with 5,233 patients, oral adjuvant chemotherapy (oral 5-FU, UFT, carmofur) was compared with observation [28]. Patients receiving oral fluoropyrimidine chemotherapy had better DFS (hazard ratio (HR) 0.85, $p = 0.001$) and superior OS (HR 0.89, $p = 0.04$) [28].

All these studies clearly show that the oral fluoropyrimidines are at least equally effective as intravenous bolus FU/LV in the adjuvant treatment of patients with colon cancer.

Oxaliplatin

The addition of oxaliplatin (LOHP) to FU/LV as adjuvant treatment for colon cancer has been investigated in two large randomized studies. In the Multicenter International Study of LOHP/5-FU/LV in the Adjuvant Treatment of Colon Cancer (MOSAIC) trial, 2,246 patients with stage II and III colon cancer were randomly assigned to 6 months of treatment with LV5FU2 (de Gramont) or identical FU/LV + LOHP 85 mg/m^2 on day 1 of every cycle (FOLFOX-4) [29]. The primary endpoint of the study was 3-year DFS. After a median follow-up of 56.2 months, DFS was significantly higher in the FOLFOX-4 group (76.4%) compared with LV5FU2 group (69.8%). The HR was 0.77 ($p < 0.001$). For the subgroup of patients with stage III colon cancer the reduction of the relapse rate was statistically significant, with an absolute difference of 8.6% (HR 0.75). A trend but no significant difference was observed in the subgroup of patients with stage II disease, with an absolute difference of 3.5% (HR 0.82%) (table 3). Four-year survival for the whole population (both stage II and III) did not reach significance, 84.9 vs. 82.9% [30]. FOLFOX-4 was a well-tolerated schedule. The all-cause mortality in the study was 0.5% in both arms. Grade III/IV neutropenia was observed in 41% of patients receiving FOLFOX-4 compared with 5% in patients receiving LV5FU2, but infections or neutropenic fever were rare. Peripheral neuropathy was observed in 92% of the patients who received FOLFOX and in 12% was grade III. This persisted in only

Table 3. Combination chemotherapy in the adjuvant treatment of patients with colon cancer

Trial	Stage	Patients	DFS, %		HR	p
			3 years	long-term follow-up		
MOSAIC						
LV5FU2	II/III	2,246	72.9	69.8[a]	0.77	<0.001
FOLFOX-4			78.2	76.4[a]		
LV5FU2	III[b]	1,347	65.3	61.0[c]	0.76	<0.005
FOLFOX-4			72.2	69.7[c]		
NSABP-C-07						
Bolus FU/FA	II/III	2,492	71.6		0.79	0.004
FLOX			76.5			
Bolus FU/FA	III[b]	1,774	65.5		0.77	NA
FLOX			72.2			
CALGB-C89803						
Bolus FU/FA	III	1,260	identical		NA	0.80
IFL						
ACCORD 2						
LV5FU2	High-risk III	400	60		1.19	NS
IF			51			
PETACC 3						
LV5FU2	III	2,111	60.3		0.89	0.091
IF			63.3			
LV5FU2	II/III[b]	3,005	66.8		0.88	0.050
IF			69.6			

DFS = Disease-free survival; HR = hazard ratio; MOSAIC = Multicenter International Study of Oxaliplatin/5-Fluorouracil/Leucovorin in the Adjuvant Treatment of Colon Cancer; LV5FU2 = leucovorin + fluorouracil de Gramont regimen; NSABP = National Surgery Adjuvant Breast and Bowel Project; FOLFOX 4 = oxaliplatin + leucovorin + fluorouracil de Gramont regimen; NA = not analyzable; CALGB = Cancer and Leukemia Group B; PETACC = Pan European Trial Adjuvant Colon Cancer; FLOX = bolus FU/FA + oxaliplatin; FA = folinic acid; IFL = FU/FA + irinotecan; IF = LV5FU2 + irinotecan.

[a] Disease-free survival with median follow-up of 56.2 months.

[b] Secondary endpoint.

[c] Four-year disease-free survival.

1.2% for 12 months and in 0.5% for 24 months. Grade II neuropathy was seen in 4% of patients at 12 months and 3% at 24 months. Grade I neuropathy was present in 22% of patients at 12 months and 14% at 24 months, showing an improvement with time for all grades peripheral neuropathy [30].

In the NSABP C-07 study, 2,492 patients were randomly assigned to a bolus schedule of FU/LV (Roswell-Park for three cycles) versus the same FU/LV schedule + LOHP (FLOX regimen is identical to FU/LV + LOHP 85 mg/m^2 on days 1, 15, 29 of each cycle) [31] (table 1). The primary endpoint of the study was 3-year DFS and it was superior for patients who received FLOX compared with FU/LV (76.5 vs. 71.6%). It corresponds to a 21% reduction in the risk of recurrence and death with the addition of LOHP. The HR for DFS was 0.79, p = 0.004. Survival data are not yet available. In total, 85.4% of patients who received FLOX regimen experienced peripheral neuropathy during treatment and 29.4% had symptoms 12 months later. Grade III neuropathy was noticed in 8% of patients during FLOX and 0.5% had grade III neuropathy at 12 months after stopping treatment. Gastrointestinal toxicity was relatively high, 38% of patients who received FLOX had grade III or IV diarrhea. Neutropenia occurred in 4% of patients treated with FLOX.

This NSABP trial confirms the increased activity of LOHP when added to FU/LV in the adjuvant treatment of colon cancer. But, until the results of C-07 are presented in full, it is premature to assume that FLOX and FOLFOX are interchangeable.

Irinotecan

Three trials comparing irinotecan/FU/LV with FU/LV have been reported. The United States Cancer and Leukemia Group B 89803 randomly assigned 1,264 patients with stage III colon cancer to bolus FU/LV (Roswell-Park schedule) versus the same FU/LV + irinotecan (IFL regimen) [32] (table 1). The study closed early because a higher treatment-related death rate was reported in the IFL arm. After a median follow-up of 2.6 years, no difference was observed between the two treatment groups regarding the DFS or OS. Therefore, IFL regimen cannot be considered as an option in the adjuvant treatment of patients with stage III colon cancer [33].

The French ACCORD 2 study compared LV5FU2 regimen with LV5FU2 + irinotecan (IF regimen) (tables 1, 3) [34] in 400 patients with high-risk stage III colon cancer. High-risk stage III was considered the disease presented with N2 or N1/N2 disease detected by occlusion or perforation. No improvement was observed in DFS (60% in patients treated with LV5FU2 versus 51% in patients treated with IF, HR 1.19) and the toxicity was higher for patients treated with IF.

The Pan European Trial Adjuvant Colon Cancer (PETACC)-3 trial was designed to search for an improvement in 3-year DFS, in 3,005 patients with stage II–III colon cancer, treated with irinotecan plus an infusional 5-FU schedule (AIO or FOLFIRI) [35] (tables 1, 3). This protocol defined that the occurrence of a new non-colorectal primary would be counted as an event in DFS, a definition not in accordance with most other adjuvant trials. The primary endpoint was 3-year DFS for patients with stage III disease. Secondary endpoints were DFS in the pooled stage II/III population, relapse-free survival (equal to DFS excluding second primaries non-colon cancers) in stage III patients, survival and safety. An imbalance was noted between the two arms: 17% of patients treated with LV5FU2 + irinotecan had T4 tumors, while 13% of patients treated with LV5FU2 had T4 tumors ($p = 0.006$), and that because there was no stratification for T stage. At a medium follow-up of 38 months the primary endpoint of the study was not met. Three-year DFS for stage III was 63.3% for patients treated with irinotecan compared with 60.3% for patients treated without irinotecan. The HR for 3-year DFS was 0.89, $p = 0.091$. DFS for the pooled population (stage II and III) was borderline significant: 69.6 vs. 66.8%, HR was 0.88, $p = 0.05$. The relapse-free survival for patients with stage III colon cancer was 66 vs. 62.2% for patients with stage II. The HR for 3-year relapse-free survival was 0.86, $p = 0.045$. Patients receiving irinotecan experienced slightly higher toxicity. The 60-day mortality was <0.5% in both arms and the mortality within 30 days of the last treatment was <1% in both arms. Based on the consistent results of these trials, one can surmise that any benefit from adjuvant irinotecan appears to be of small magnitude and not likely clinically relevant when given on current FU/LV schedules.

Other Drugs

Two ongoing European trials have been designed to evaluate the addition of drugs other than LOHP or irinotecan in the adjuvant treatment of colon cancer. The Groupe Régionale d'Etudes du Cancer Colorectal (GERCOR)-03 study compares the impact of DFS on one of four containing arms: chronomodulated FU/LV with and without carboplatin or infusional FU/LV with and without carboplatin. The second study, PETACC-5, investigates whether the addition of celecoxib to FU/LV will improve DFS over placebo in 1,450 randomized patients with stage III colon cancer (table 4).

Biologics

Cetuximab is a chimeric monoclonal antibody targeting the epidermal growth factor receptor and is active in metastatic setting in patients with irinotecan refractory disease either alone or in combination with irinotecan [36]. Non-randomized phase II studies shared promising results in a first-line setting when cetuximab was combined with FOLFOX or FOLFIRI. Large studies have been designed and are ongoing in Europe and in USA in the adjuvant treatment of colon cancer evaluating FOLFOX with or without cetuximab (protocols N0147 and PETACC-8) (table 4).

Bevacizumab is a humanized monoclonal antibody that targets vascular endothelial growth factor, which is essential for tumor angiogenesis. In randomized trials for metastatic colon cancer, the addition of bevacizumab to irinotecan/FU/LV in first-line treatments or to LOHP/FU/LV in second-line treatments have shown increased activity [37]. In the adjuvant setting, two large trials are ongoing for patients with stage II/III colon cancer. The AVANT trial plans to randomize 3,450 patients with high-risk stage II and stage III colon cancer to receive FOLFOX or FOLFOX + bevacizumab or XELOX + bevacizumab (table 4). The NSABP-CO8 study plans to ran-

Table 4. Ongoing phase III trials of adjuvant therapy for colon cancer

Trial	Chemotherapy regimen	Stage	Anticipated enrollment, n	Primary endpoint
NSABP C-08	Arm 1: FOLFOX Arm 2: FOLFOX + bevacizumab	II, III	2,632	DFS
NCCTG N0147	Arm 1: FOLFOX Arm 2: FOLFOX + cetuximab	III	2,300	OS
ECOG 5202	Arm 1: FOLFOX Arm 2: FOLFOX + bevacizumab Arm 3: Observation (low-risk)	II	3,610; 1,200 high-risk	3-year DFS
GERCOR-03	Arm 1: Chromo 5-FU/LV ± carboplatin Arm 2: INF 5-FU/LV ± carboplatin	IIB, III	660–800	DFS
EORTC 40023/PETACC5	Arm 1: 5-FU/LV + 3 years' celecoxib Arm 2: 5-FU/LV + 3 years' placebo	III	1,450	DFS
AVANT	Arm 1: FOLFOX Arm 2: FOLFOX + bevacizumab Arm 3: XELOX + bevacizumab	II, III	3,450	DFS, OS
ACCORD-I	Arm 1: FOLFOX Arm 2: FOLFOX + cetuximab	III		

5-FU = 5-Fluorouracil; Chromo = chronomodulated; DFS = disease-free survival; EORTC = European Organization for Research and Treatment of Cancer; GERCOR = Groupe Régional d'Etudes du Cancer Colorectal; INF = infusional; LV = leucovorin; NCCTG = North Central Cancer Treatment Group; NSABP = National Surgery Adjuvant Breast and Bowel Project; OS = overall survival; PETACC = Pan European Treatment Adjuvant Colon Cancer.

domize 2,500 patients with resected stage II/III colon cancer between FOLFOX or FOLFOX + bevacizumab.

All these studies with cetuximab and bevacizumab in the adjuvant setting are designed to significantly improve 3-year DFS in patients with resected stage II/III colon cancer, and the oncology community anxiously awaits the results of these trials to see if the biologic agents will have the same impact on DFS and OS in the adjuvant setting as they have shown in metastatic disease.

Intraperitoneal-Intraportal Chemotherapy

Besides intravenous chemotherapy, several studies have investigated the role of chemotherapy either intraperitoneally or intraportally. Large randomized studies could not show a better outcome for patients treated with system 5-FU-based chemotherapy in combination with intraportal or intraperitoneal chemotherapy as adjuvant treatment [38].

Adjuvant Treatment for Stage II Colon Cancer

The therapeutic approach in stage II colon cancer is more controversial because of the lack of a large number of prospective randomized trials. Most of the data derive from prospectively defined subgroup analyses of trials that include stage II and stage III patients with colon cancer. The result pooled analyses as well as the Quick And Simple And Reliable (QUASAR)-1 study have attempted to answer that question [25, 39–41]. All these analyses confirm a relative risk reduction of death of 20% (12–30%) provided by adjuvant 5-FU-based chemotherapy in patients with stage II disease, but the confidence intervals are wide and do not allow definite conclusions of true benefit. In a subset analysis of the MOSAIC trial, the proportional benefit of LOHP over FU/LV and the relative risk reduction of DFS of 20% remained the same for stage II and stage III patients [42]. Whether adjuvant chemotherapy improves outcomes in stage II colon cancer patients is unlikely to ever be quantified as the number of patients needed is very high (approximately 4,000 patients per arm). However, the true absolute 5-year survival benefit from adjuvant treatment for stage II colon cancer is likely between 2 and 4% [43] and may be higher with the newer agents. The most important ongoing clinical trial for stage II disease is ECOG 5202. This study aims to enroll 3,600 stage II patients. Tumors will be tested for loss of heterozygosity 18q and microsatellite instability. Patients with high-risk tumors (both loss of heterozygosity and microsatellite stability) will be randomized to FOLFOX or to FOFLFOX with bevacizumab. The low-risk stage II patients will be followed prospectively as an observation arm. The tumor blocks and blood from the low-risk cohort of patients will be analyzed in a translational program in order to evaluate known and possible new prognostic and predictive markers.

Future Directions

The active new drugs have led to new and more questions in the field of adjuvant chemotherapy for CRC and the answers to these questions can be given through large, well-designed, randomized trials. At the 2004 ASCO Meeting, a report correlated closely 3-year DFS with 5-year OS. Following this report, at the 2005 ASCO Meeting, the same authors announced that 2-year DFS is also tightly correlated with 5-year OS (correlation coefficient 0.74). Two-year DFS is a very attractive endpoint, but it would be premature to base studies only on this endpoint without further follow-up. If it becomes true, these surrogates will lead to more rapid reporting of adjuvant outcomes and shorten the waiting time for new effective regimens to reach the community.

Many questions regarding the selection of patients for aggressive adjuvant chemotherapy remain unanswered. Three classes of factors could be useful in clinical decision-making: stage-independent prognostic factors, factors that can predict response to treatment and factors that can predict toxicity to various agents. Stage-independent prognostic factors could be used to distinguish a group of patients at higher risk than similarly staged patients, so that they receive more aggressive treatment. ECOG 5202 trial uses 18qLOH (loss of heterozygosity) and MSS (microsatellite stability) as bad prognostic factors. In patients with stage II colon cancer, 18qLOH carries risk of recurrence that is more akin to patients with stage III at presentation [44]. Microsatellite instability (MSI) carries a lesser risk of later metastatic recurrence that does an MSS tumor phenotype [45]. Factors that can predict response to treatment could help select which treatment option is most likely to be beneficial. MSI is considered to be a predictor of response to 5-FU-based adjuvant chemotherapy, as it results from some retrospective analyses but not by others [46–48]. Prospective studies are needed to confirm the ability of high MSI expression in predicting response to 5-FU-based chemotherapy. Another factor that could be useful in predicting 5-FU response is high thymidylate synthase (TS) expression, which correlates with low chance of response to 5-FU, as results retrospectively from many studies. The expression of TS may not be of great clinical utility, because 5-FU may be a requirement for LOHP efficacy and not dispensable even in high TS patients. Pharmacogenomics predict toxicity by testing for common genetic polymorphism in the 5-FU-inactivating enzyme dihydropyrimidine dehydrogenase (DPD), activity and severe, potentially lethal, 5-FU toxicity. A cheap and easily reproducible method for testing for this abnormality is sought after, so that 5-FU alternatives might be chosen in patients with very low DPD activity. Another useful predictor of toxicity is polymorphism of the UGT1A1 gene, which is responsible for glucuronidation and thus inactivation of SN-38, the active metabolite of irinotecan, and predicts for severe neutropenia in irinotecan administration [49].

Summary and Conclusion

The 1980s introduced clinical trials that showed for the first time the effectiveness of adjuvant chemotherapy for patients with resected stage III colon cancer. Since the establishment of 5-FU + levamisole in adjuvant treatment, many large randomized trials have modified adjuvant chemotherapy, showing that: 6 months of 5-FU/LV is equivalent to 1 year of 5-FU/levamisole; weekly schedules of 5-FU/LV are equivalent to the monthly schedule; levamisole is not necessary in the adjuvant therapy; the high-dose 5-FU/LV is equivalent to the low dose with different toxicity profiles, and infusional 5-FU schedules are equivalent to bolus 5-FU schedules with less toxicity. In more recent studies, oral fluoropyrimidines (UFT and capecitabine) are proven to be of equal efficacy with bolus 5-FU/LV, IFL is more toxic and not superior to bolus 5-FU/LV. Pending data will determine the efficacy of FOLFIRI compared to 5-FU/LV. Combinations of oral agents with LOHP are being studied and trials that have incorporated the new monoclonal antibodies cetuximab and bevacizumab are ongoing. Current strategies in investigation of the effects of adjuvant chemotherapy include prospective analysis of prognostic and predictive markers of risk and response.

References

1 GLOBOCAN: Cancer Incidence Mortality and Prevalence Worldwide. Version IARC CancerBase No 5. Lyon, IARC Press, 2001.

2 Obrand DI, Gordon PH: Incidence and pattern of recurrence following curative resection for colorectal carcinoma. Dis Colon Rectum 1997;40:15–24.

3 American Joint Committee on Cancer: Cancer Staging Manual, ed 6. New York, Springer, 2002.

4 Sashiro S: Recurrence pattern after curative resection of colorectal cancer in patients followed for a minimum of 10 years. Hepatogastroenterology 2003;50:1362–1366.

5 Sargent DJ, Wieand S, Benedeui J, et al: Disease-free survival vs. overall survival as a primary endpoint for adjuvant colon cancer studies. Individual patient data from 12,915 patients on 15 randomized trials. J Clin Oncol 2004;22(suppl):245, abstr 3502.

6 Wolmark N, Fischer B, Rockette H, et al: Postoperative adjuvant chemotherapy or BCG for colon cancer: results from NSABP C-01. J Natl Cancer Inst 1988;80:30–36.

7 Laurie JA, Moertel CG, Fleming TR, et al: Surgical adjuvant therapy of large-bowel carcinoma: an evaluation of levamisole and the combination of levamisole and fluorouracil. The North Central Treatment Group and the Mayo Clinic. J Clinic Oncol 1989;7: 1447–1456.

8 Windle R, Bell PR, Shaw D: Five-year results of a randomized trial of adjuvant 5-fluorouracil and levamisole in colorectal cancer. Br J Surg 1987;74:569–572.

9 Moertel CG, Fleming TR, Macdonald JS, et al: Levamisole and fluorouracil for adjuvant therapy of resected colon carcinoma. N Engl J Med 1990;322:352–358.

10 Moertel CG, Fleming TR, Macdonald JS, et al: Fluorouracil + levamisole as effective adjuvant therapy after resection of stage III colon carcinoma: a final report. Ann Intern Med 1995;122:321–326.

11 Francini G, Petrioli R, Lorenzini L, et al: Folinic acid and 5-fluorouracil as adjuvant chemotherapy in colon cancer. Gastroenterology 1994;106:899–906.

12 O'Connell MJ, Mailliard JA, Kahn MJ, et al: Controlled trial of fluorouracil and low-dose leucovorin given for 6 months as postoperative adjuvant therapy for colon cancer. J Clin Oncol 1997;15:246–250.

13 International Multicentre Pooled Analysis of Colon Cancer Trials (IMPACT) Investigators: Efficacy of adjuvant fluorouracil and folinic acid in colon cancer. Lancet 1995;345: 939.

14 Taal BG, Van Tinteren H, Zoetmulder FA: Adjuvant 5-FU + levamisole in colonic or rectal cancer: improved survival in stage II and III. Br J Cancer 2001;85:1437–1443.

15 O'Connell MJ, Laurie JA, Kahn M, et al: Prospectively randomized trial of postoperative adjuvant chemotherapy in patients with high-risk colon cancer. J Clin Oncol 1998;16: 295–300.

16 Wolmark N, Rockette H, Fisher B, et al: The benefit of leucovorin-modulated fluorouracil as postoperative adjuvant therapy for primary colon cancer: results from National Surgical Breast and Bowel Project C-03. J Clinic Oncol 1993;11:1879–1887.

17 Wolmark N, Rockette H, Mamounas E, et al: Clinical trial to assess the relative efficacy of fluorouracil and leucovorin, fluorouracil and levamisole, and fluorouracil, leucovorin, and levamisole in patients with Dukes' B and C carcinoma of the colon: results from the National Surgical Breast and Bowel Project C-04. J Clin Oncol 1999;17:3533–3559.

18 Wolmark N, Bryant J, Smith R, et al: Adjuvant 5-fluorouracil and leucovorin with or without interferon alfa-2a in colon carcinoma: Surgical Breast and Bowel Project C-05. J Natl Cancer Inst 1998;90:1810–1816.

19 QUASAR Collaborative Group: Comparison of fluorouracil with additional levamisole, higher-dose folinic acid, or both, as adjuvant chemotherapy for colorectal cancer: a randomized trial. Lancet 2000;355:1588–1596.

20 Porschen R, Bermann A, Loffler T, et al: Fluorouracil + leucovorin as effective adjuvant chemotherapy in curatively resected stage III colon cancer: results of the trial adjCCA-01. J Clin Oncol 2001;19:1787–1794.

21 Haller DG, Catalano PJ, MacDonald JS, Mayer RJ: Fluorouracil, leucovorin and levamisole adjuvant therapy for colon cancer: five-year final report of Int-0089. Proc Am Soc Clin Oncol 1998;17:256A.

22 Andre T, Colin P, Louvet C, et al: Semimonthly versus monthly regimen of fluorouracil and leucovorin administered for 24 or 36 weeks as adjuvant therapy in stage II and III colon cancer. J Clin Oncol 2003;21:2896–2903.

23 Poplin EA, Benedetti JK, Estes NC, et al: Phase III Southwest Oncology Group 9415/ Intergroup 0153 randomized trial of fluorouracil, leucovorin, and levamisole versus fluorouracil continuous infusion, and levamisole for adjuvant treatment of stage III and high-risk stage II colon cancer. J Clin Oncol 2005;23:1819–1825.

24 Andre T, Quinaux E, Louvet C, et al: Updated results at 6 years of the GERCOR C96. 1. A phase III study comparing LV5FU2 to monthly 5-FU-leucovorin as adjuvant treatment for Dukes' B2 and C colon cancer patients (abstract). J Clin Oncol 2005;23:250S.

25 Gill S, Loprinzi CL, Sargent DJ, et al: Pooled analysis of fluorouracil-based adjuvant therapy for stage II and III colon cancer: Who benefits and by how much? J Clin Oncol 2004;22:1797–1806.

26 Twelves C, Wond A, Nowacki M, et al: Capecitabine as adjuvant treatment for stage III colon cancer. N Engl J Med 2005;352: 2696–2704.

27 Wolmark N, Wieand S, Lembersky B, et al: A phase III trial comparing oral UFT to FULV in stage II and III carcinoma of the colon: results of NSABP Protocol C-06. Proc Am Soc Clin Oncol 2004;22:247S.

28 Sakamoto J, Ohashi Y, Hamada C, et al: Efficacy of oral adjuvant therapy after resection of colorectal cancer: 5-year results from thee randomized trials. J Clin Oncol 2004; 22:484–492.

29 Andre T, Boni C, Mounedji-BoudiafL, et al: Oxaliplatin, fluorouracil and leucovorin as adjuvant treatment for colon cancer. N Engl J Med 2004;350:2343–2351.

30 De Gramont A, Boni C, Navarro M, et al: Oxaliplatin/5-FU/LV in the adjuvant treatment of stage II and III colon cancer: efficacy results with a median follow-up of 4 years. J Clin Oncol 2005;23:246S.

31 Wolmark N, Wieand SH, Kuebler J, et al: A phase III trial comparing FULV + oxaliplatin in stage II or II carcinoma of the colon: results of NSABP protocol C-07. J Clin Oncol 2005;23:246S.

32 Rothenberg M, Meropol N, Poplin E, et al: Mortality associated with irinotecan + bolus fluorouracil/leucovorin: summary findings of an independent panel. J Clin Oncol 2001; 19:3801–3807.

33 Saltz L, Niedwiecki D, Hollis D, et al: Irinotecan + fluorouracil/leucovorin versus fluorouracil/leucovorin in stage III colon cancer (intergroup trial CALGB C89903). J Clin Oncol 2004;22:245S.

34 Ychou M, Raoul JL, Douillard JY, et al: A phase III randomized trial of LV5FU2 + CP-11 vs. LV5FU2 alone in adjuvant high risk colon cancer (FNCLCC Accord02/FFCD9802). J Clin Oncol 2005;23:246S.

35 Van Custem E, Labianca D, Hossfeld D, et al: Randomized phase III trial comparing infused irinotecan/5-fluorouracil/folinic acid vs. 5-FU/FA in stage III colon cancer patients. J Clin Oncol 2005;23:LBA8.

36 Cunningham D, Humblet Y, Siena S, et al: Cetuximab monotherapy and cetuximab + irinotecan in irinotecan-refractory metastatic colorectal cancer. N Engl J Med 2004; 351:337–345.

37 Hurwitz H, Fehrenbacher L, Novotny W, et al: Bevacizumab + irinotecan, fluorouracil, and leucovorin for metastatic colorectal cancer. N Engl J Med 2004;350:2335–2342.

38 Nordlinger B, Rougier P, Arnaud JC, et al: Adjuvant regional chemotherapy and systemic chemotherapy versus systemic chemotherapy alone in patients with stage II-III colorectal cancer: a multicentre randomized controlled phase III trial. Lancet Oncol 2005; 6:459–468.

39 Mamounas E, Wieand S, Wolmark N, et al: Comparative efficacy of adjuvant chemotherapy in patients with Dukes' C colon cancer: results from four National Surgical Adjuvant Breast and Bowel Project adjuvant studies (C-01, C-02, C-03, and C-04). J Clin Oncol 1999;17:1349–1355.
40 International Multicentre Pooled Analysis of B2 Colon Cancer Trials (IMPACT B2) Investigators: Efficacy of adjuvant fluorouracil and folinic acid in B2 colon cancer. J Clin Oncol 1999;17:1356–1363.
41 Gray RG, Barnwell J, Hills R, et al: QUASAR a randomized study of adjuvant chemotherapy vs. observation including 3,238 colorectal cancer patients (abstract). Proc Am Soc Clin Oncol 2004;22:3501.
42 Hickish T, Boni M, Navarro M, et al: FOLFOX-4 as adjuvant treatment for stage II colon cancer: subpopulation data from the MOSAIC trial (abstract). Proc Am Soc Clin Oncol 2004;23:275.
43 Benson AB, Schrag D, Somerfield MR, et al: American Society of Clinical Oncology recommendations on adjuvant chemotherapy for stage II colon cancer. J Clin Oncol 2004; 22:3408–3419.
44 Fearon ER, Cho KR, Nigro JM, et al: Identification of a chromosome 18q gene that is altered in colorectal cancers. Science 1990;247: 49–56.
45 Gryfe R, Kim H, Hsieh ET, et al: Tumor microsatellite instability and clinical outcome in young patients with colorectal cancer. N Engl J Med 2000;342:69–77.
46 Elsaleh H, Shannon B, Iacopetta B: Microsatellite instability as a molecular marker for very good survival in colorectal cancer patients receiving adjuvant chemotherapy. Gastroenterology 2001;120:1309–1310.
47 Elsaleh H, Iacopetta B: Microsatellite instability is a predictive marker for survival benefit from adjuvant chemotherapy in a population-based series of stage III colorectal carcinoma. Clin Colorectal Cancer 2001;1: 104–109.
48 Ribic CM, Sargent DJ, Moore MJ, et al: Tumor microsatellite-instability status as predictor of from fluorouracil-based adjuvant chemotherapy for colon cancer. N Engl J Med 2003;349:247–257.
49 Iyer L, Das S, Janisch L, et al: UGT1A1*28 polymorphism as a determinant of irinotecan disposition and toxicity. Pharmacogenomics J 2002;2:43–47.

Review Article

Digestive Diseases

Dig Dis 2007;25:76–79
DOI: 10.1159/000099173

Early Rectal Cancer: Definition and Management

Emanuele Lezoche[a] Maddalena Baldarelli[b] Angelo De Sanctis[b]
Giovanni Lezoche[a] Mario Guerrieri[b]

[a]Department of Surgery 'Paride Stefanini', II Clinica Chirurgica, University 'La Sapienza', Rome, and
[b]Department of General Surgery, University of Ancona, 'Umberto I' Hospital, Ancona, Italy

Key Words
Rectal cancer · Preoperative staging · Preoperative radiotherapy and chemotherapy · Transanal endoscopic microsurgery

Abstract
Background: Local excision of rectal cancer is an alternative to radical resection but today its role surrounding the management of patients with early stage rectal cancer (T1-T2-N0) represents an important surgical issue. ***Aim:*** To analyze the results of 135 patients with early stage low rectal cancer treated with local excision by transanal endoscopic microsurgery and in the case of T2 also by neoadjuvant therapy. ***Study Design:*** 135 patients with T1-T2-N0-M0 rectal cancer were enrolled in the study. Staging according to the definitive histological findings was as follows: pT0 in 24 patients (17.8%), pT1 in 66 patients (48.8%) and pT2 in 45 patients (33.4%). ***Results:*** Minor complications were observed in 12 patients (8.8%) whereas major complications were seen only in 2 patients (1.5%). At a median follow-up of 78 (36–125) months, local recurrences occurred in 4 patients and distal metastasis in 2 patients (all patients were staged preoperatively T2). Disease-free survival rates in T1 and T2 patients were 100 and 93% respectively at the end of follow-up. ***Conclusions:*** With respect to local recurrence and survival rate, the long-term results of early stage rectal cancer in patients treated with transanal endoscopic microsurgery were similar to those reported in the literature after conventional surgery (total mesorectal excision).

Colorectal cancer is the second most common cause of cancer deaths in the Western world. More than 35,000 new rectal cancers are diagnosed every year in the USA and 25% are stage I disease. Fewer than half of these cases are lesions confined to the mucosa and submucosa [1].

In the past the gold standard of treatment for all low rectal cancers was anterior resection with coloanal or low rectal anastomosis and abdominoperinal resection. These procedures led to good results in terms of local recurrence and 5-year survival rate [1–4]. Unfortunately, resection of the rectum is a major surgery procedure associated with significant morbidity (7–68%), mortality (0–6.5%), alteration in body image and sometimes distressing functional consequences for the patients [2].

In the past the use of local excision was limited to high-risk patients for major surgery, especially in the elderly and those who refused radical surgery because of permanent colostomy. However, the high number of complications, functional sequels and sphincter sacrifice rates associated with radical resection prompted researchers to reevaluate local excision for distal rectal cancer as an al-

KARGER

Fax +41 61 306 12 34
E-Mail karger@karger.ch
www.karger.com

0257–2753/07/0251–0076$23.50/0

Accessible online at:
www.karger.com/ddi

Emanuele Lezoche
Department of Surgery 'Paride Stefanini'
II Clinica Chirurgica, University 'La Sapienza'
Viale del Policlinico, IT–00161 Rome (Italy)
Tel. +39 06 4997 8851, Fax +39 06 4997 8849, E-Mail emanuele.lezoche@uniroma1.it

ternative to radical resection. Excision has been suggested as a possible curative therapy.

Recent literature considers local excision as curative surgery in most of the patients with a primary tumor which is limited to the mucosa and submucosa (T1-N0-M0) and does not present cytological or histological high-risk features such as poorly differentiated cells, vascular and neural invasion, presence of mucinous histology and tumor ulceration) [5–9]. In these patients, local excision of rectal tumors preserves anal continence, bladder and sexual functions and achieves the same oncological results. In T1 patients, local excision is feasible because the curative rate is high (>90/95%) and the risk of recurrence is low (<10/5%) as reported in the literature [1, 4].

Winde et al. [5] reported an important study where they compared the results of local excision for early rectal carcinomas using transanal endoscopic microsurgery versus anterior resection. They concluded that the results were comparable in local recurrence and survival rates and that the TEM technique should be preferred because of the superior overview during operation and for the full-thickness excision.

Today, the role of local excision combined with new adjuvant therapy in the management of patients with T2-N0 rectal cancer represents an issue of debate. Once the tumor invades the muscularis propria (T2), preoperative radiochemotherapy is strongly recommended because local excision alone has a too high percentage of local recurrence [4, 6]. Data, especially from Europe, have suggested that preoperative radiation reduces local recurrence rates and improves overall survival when compared with surgery alone, and that it is more effective than postoperative radiotherapy [2–4, 7–19]. Therefore, high-dose preoperative radiation offers the opportunity for a downstage or a reduction in the neoplastic mass in order to preserve the anal sphincter and enhance quality of life postoperatively. The advantages of preoperative new adjuvant therapy are: biological (decreased tumor seeding at the time of surgery, lymph node sterilization of micrometastasis and increased radiosensitivity due to more oxygenated cells) and functional aspects (ability to change the coloanal resection to local excision). An additional benefit in patients with local advanced and unresectable disease is the possibility to increase the resectability rate [20–23].

Many surgical options are described in the literature for local therapy of rectal cancer such as transanal and transsphincteric approaches. Transanal excision (Parks, Mason, Francillon, etc.) is the most popular technique: it has very low complications rates (0–15%) and early recovery but, for technical reasons, this method is limited to low and mid-rectal lesions and it does not allow an adequate view of the operative field and is generally performed as a full-thickness excision without a complete ablation of the local perirectal fat [6]. Other approaches of local excision for rectal cancer such as the transsphincteric or transsacral approach have been described. These techniques can reach higher lesions, but have high complication rates up to 40% of cases and only few studies including a small number of patients of local excision have been reported [6].

In 1983, Buess et al. in Germany developed transanal endoscopic microsurgery (TEM) [24], and resolved many problems of traditionally local treatment. This method is a minimally invasive technique, has a great magnification and an excellent lighting of the operative field that allows a clear identification of the margins of the lesion and the precise excision of tumors in the rectum extending into the upper rectum or lower sigmoid colon via the transanal approach. Compared with the traditional transanal approach using Park's retractor, TEM allows an excellent exposure of the operative field with a stereoscopic endoscopic vision that permits to perform a complete full-thickness excision with an appropriate margin (ablation with 1 cm of surrounding free margin) and to remove all the adjacent perirectal fat making the same plane of dissection utilized in the TME (the so-called 'holy plane'). The precise excision of the tumor performed by TEM facilitates a more accurate and oncologically correct excision, in fact the resection margin of the local surgical specimen is of critical importance in relation to the development of recurrence.

Selection of appropriate patients for local excision is a crucial step [2]. Due to the fact that local excision of rectal cancer does not remove the draining lymph nodes, only cancers localized on the rectal wall are suitable for curative local excision alone. Patient selection needs to be based on the probability of nodal disease. Accurate preoperative assessment of depth of invasion is important because the risk of lymph node metastases increases with T-stage being 0–12% for T1, 12–28% for T2, and 36–79 for T3–T4 lesions [24]. Thus, preoperative T-staging and the exclusion of distant metastases are mandatory for an appropriate selection of patients eligible for curative local excision. Therefore, the preoperative staging must include: digital examination, endoscopy, endosonography (EUS) and computed tomography (CT) and/or magnetic resonance imaging (MRI). Clinical examination by digital rectal examination is the usual method of staging distal and mid-rectal cancer, but the accuracy depends on the experience of the examiner. The most useful adjunct for the preoperative assessment of rectal lesions is EUS that allows clear visualization of the layers of the rectal wall and thus enables the depth of invasion to be measured accurately. EUS, although operator-dependent, can be performed with minimal bowel preparation and patient discomfort, and it is currently considered the most accurate method for local staging of rectal cancer. EUS has an 82–93% accuracy with respect to depth of invasion, although overstaging has been reported [24]. Assessment of lymph node involvement is less reliable, with reported accuracy of 65–81% [24]. Metastatic lymph nodes can be differentiated from reactive changes because they are hypoechoic and irregular. The vast majority of patients with rectal cancer have an abdominopelvic CT prior to surgery in order to explore the lymph node status and to identify metastatic disease. MRI, when used, has accuracy rates comparable to CT scan. In our experience the best diagnostic tool to evaluate the T-staging for low rectal lesion is the transanal EUS with a rotative probe of 7 MHz; MRI and CT give a more accurate evaluation of the N. Recently the introduction in clinical practice of ultrasound with fine-needle biopsy, multislide spiral CT scan and so-called 'virtual endoscopy' have significantly improved our ability to achieve a correct preoperative staging of rectal cancer.

In conclusion, local excision can be considered as curative in patients with a primary tumor confined to the mucosa and submucosa (T1N0M0), without high-risk features; on the contrary, once the tumor invades the muscularis propria (T2) neoadjuvant treatment is strongly recommended if we are planning to perform local excision in order to avoid the risk of a major operation.

Personal Experience

516 patients underwent TEM surgery at the Departments of Surgery 'Paride Stefanini' (II Clinica Chirurgica, University of Rome 'La Sapienza') and General Surgery of the University of Ancona from May 1992 to December 2005: 306 (59.3%) for adenomas, 196 (38%) for rectal carcinomas and 14 (2.7%) for other miscellaneous rectal lesions. 135 (26.2%) patients (92 male and 43 women) were treated by TEM for T1-T2-N0-M0 rectal cancers (51 patients T1-N0-M0 and 84 patients T2-N0-M0). Mean age was of 63 (range 31–95) years.

The preoperative staging was evaluated by: total colonoscopy, standard endoscopic biopsies (taken at 1 cm around the tumor and identified with a number), rigid rectoscopy (in order to perform the macrobiopsies of the tumor area, to measure the exact distance of the lesion from the anal verge to evaluate the circumferential tumor localization and to select the position of the patient on the surgical table during the operation), transanal EUS, MRI and/or CT, bone scintigraphy, chest X-rays and digital examination to evaluate tumor fixation.

Patients with preoperative diagnosis of T2 rectal cancer underwent preoperative radiotherapy according the technique described by Marks et al. [21–23]. The total dose given was 50.4 Gy in 28 fractions over 5 weeks. The irradiated areas were: anus, rectum, mesorectum, regional and iliac lymph nodes. Continuous infusion of 5-FU, 200 $mg/m^2/day$, was performed as long as radiotherapy treatment lasted.

Forty days after the end of neoadjuvant therapy a new preoperative evaluation of the lesion and staging was performed by endoscopy to determine the tumor diameter changing (using as reference point the tattoo spots), transanal ultrasound, CT scan and/or MRI and digital examination. The operations were performed about 45–55 days after the end of radiochemotherapy.

Results

Minor complications occurred in 12 patients (8.8%) and included a partially leaking suture in 9 (6.6%) patients, stool incontinence in 2 (1.5%) cases, and rectal hemorrhage in 1 (0.7%) patient. We observed major complications only in 2 patients (1.5%). Definitive histology in the T1 group confirmed pT1 in all patients. In T2 patients, histology demonstrated 24 pT0, 15 pT1 and 45 pT2.

Average follow-up was 63 (range 3–164) months. Neither recurrence nor cancer-related mortality was observed in pT0 and pT1 rectal cancer patients. Local failure occurred in 4 pT2 patients after 30, 12, 8 and 6 months respectively and all patients underwent laparoscopic abdominal perineal resection. The first patient died from systemic diffusion of the tumor 4 months after reoperation, the second patient had a recurrence after 12 months of follow-up and underwent laparoscopic abdominoperineal resection and later died from systemic neoplastic disease, while the other 2 patients are still alive and disease-free. Two pT2 patients developed metastasis: the first underwent hepatic resection and died 13 months later from systemic disease and the second died 24 months later from hepatic and lung metastasis. At the end of follow-up, specific rectal survival was 100% for T1 patients and 93% for T2 patients. Overall survival was 94.1% for T1 and 88.1% for T2.

References

1 Blair S, Ellenhorn JD: Transanal excision for low rectal cancers is curative in early-stage disease with favorable histology. Am Surg 2000;66:817–820.

2 Nastro P, Beral D, Hartley J, Monson JRT: Local excision of rectal cancer: review of literature. Dig Surg 2005;22:6–15.

3 Chakravarti A, Compton CC, Shellito PC, Wood WC, Landry J, Machuta SR, et al: Long-term follow-up of patients with rectal cancers managed by local excision with and without adjuvant irradiation. Ann Surg 1999;239:49–54.

4 Kim CJ, Yeatman TJ, Coppola D, Trotti A, Williams B, Barthel JS, Dinwoodie W, Karl RC, Marcet J: Local excision of T2 and T3 rectal cancers after downstaging chemoradiation. Ann Surg 2001;234:352–359.

5 Winde G, Nottberg H. Keller R, et al: Surgical cure for early rectal carcinomas (T1). Transanal endoscopic microsurgery vs. anterior resection. Dis Colon Rectum 1996;39:969–976.

6 Sengupta S, Tjandra JJ: Local excision of rectal cancer. What is the evidence? Dis Colon Rectum 2001;44:1345–1361.

7 Heintz A, Morschel M, Junginger T: Comparison of results after transanal endoscopic microsurgery and radical resection for T1 carcinoma of the rectum. Surg Endosc 1998; 12:1145–1148.

8 Varma MG, Rogers SJ, Schrock TR, Welton ML: Local excision of rectal carcinoma. Arch Surg 1999;134:863–868.

9 Neary P, Makin GB, White TJ, White E, Hartley J, MacDonald A, Lee PWR, Monson JRT: Transanal endoscopic microsurgery: a viable operative alternative in selected patients with rectal lesions. Ann Surg Oncol 2003;10:1106–1111.

10 Bozzetto F, Baratti D, Andreola S, Zucali R, Schiavo M, Spinelli P, Gronchi A, Bertario L, Mariani L, Gennari L: Preoperative radiation therapy for patients with T2-T3 carcinoma of the middle-to-lower rectum. Cancer 1999;86:398–404.

11 Rouanet P, Fabre JM, Dubois JB, et al: Conservative surgery for low rectal carcinoma after high-dose radiation. Ann Surg 1995; 221:67–73.

12 Habr-Gama A, Perez RO, Kiss DR, Rawet V, Scanavini A, Santinho PM, Nadalin W: Preoperative chemoradiation therapy for low rectal cancer. Impact on downstaging and sphincter-saving operations. Hepatogastroenterology 2004;51:1703–1707.

13 Lee W, Lee D, Choi S, Chun H: Transanal endoscopic microsurgery and radical surgery for T1 and T2 rectal cancer. Surg Endosc 2003;17:1283–1287.

14 Marijnem CA, Glimelius B: The role of radiotherapy in rectal cancer. Eur J Cancer 2002;38:943–952.

15 Ruo L, Guillem JG, Minsky BD, Quan SH, Paty PB, Cohen AM: Preoperative radiation with or without chemotherapy and full-thickness transanal excision for selected T2 and T3 distal rectal cancers. Int J Colorectal Dis 2002;17:54–58.

16 Martling AL, Holm T, Rutqvist LE, Moran BJ, Heald RJ, Cedemark B: Effect of surgical training programme on outcome of rectal cancer in the County of Stockholm. Stockholm Colorectal Cancer Study Group, Basingstoke Bowel Cancer Research Project. Lancet 2000;356:93–96.

17 Rodel C, Martus P, Papadoupolos T, Fuzesi L, Klimpfinger M, Fietkau R, Hohenberger W, Raab R, Sauer R, Wittekind C: Prognostic significance of tumor regression after chemoradiotherapy for rectal cancer. J Clin Oncol 2005;23:8688–8696.

18 Schell SR, Zlotecki RA, Mendenhall WM, Marsh RW, Vauyhey JN, Copeland EM III: Transanal excision of locally advanced rectal cancers downstaged using neoadjuvant chemoradiotherapy. J Am Coll Surg 2002; 194:584–591.

19 Lezoche E, Guerrieri M, Paganini AM, Baldarelli M, De Sanctis A, lezoche G: Long-term results in patients with T2-3 N0 distal rectal cancer undergoing radiotherapy before transanal endoscopic microsurgery. Br J Surg 2005;92:1546–1552.

20 Vecchio FM, Valentini V, Minsky BD, Padula GD, Venkatraman ES, Balducci M, Micciche F, Ricci R, Morgani AG, Gambacorta MA, Maurizi F, Coco C: The relationship of pathologic tumor regression grade and outcomes after preoperative therapy in rectal cancer. Int J Radiat Oncl Biol Phys 2005;62: 752–760.

21 Marks G, Mohiuddin M, Masoni L: The reality of radical sphincter preservation surgery for rectal of the distal 3 cm of rectum following high-dose radiation. Int J Radiat Oncol Biol Phys 1993;27:779–83.

22 Marks G, Mohiuddin M, Rakinic J: New hope and promise for sphincter preservation in the management of cancer of the rectum. Semin Oncol 1991;18:88–98.

23 Marks G, Mohiuddin M, Masoni L, Pecchioli L: High-dose preoperative radiation and full-thickness local excision. A new option for patients with select cancers of the rectum. Dis Colon Rectum 1990;33:735–739.

24 Balch GC, De Meo A, Guillem JG: Modern management of rectal cancer. A 2006 update. World J Gastroenterol 2006;12:3186–3195.

Original Article

Digestive Diseases

Dig Dis 2007;25:80–85
DOI: 10.1159/000099174

Conventional CT for the Prediction of an Involved Circumferential Resection Margin in Primary Rectal Cancer

Steven V.R.C. Wolberink[a, g] Regina G.H. Beets-Tan[b] Danielle F.M. de Haas-Kock[c] Mark M. Span[e] Eric J. van de Jagt[d] Cornelis J.H. van de Velde[f] Theo Wiggers[a, g]

[a]Department of Surgery, University Medical Center Groningen, Groningen; [b]Department of Radiology, University Hospital Maastricht; [c]Department of Radiation Oncology (MAASTRO), Research Institute GROW, University Hospital Maastricht, Maastricht; [d]Department of Radiology, University Medical Center Groningen; [e]Office for Medical Technology Assessment, Groningen, and [f]Department of Surgery, Leiden University Medical Center, Leiden; [g]Department of Radiology, Onze Lieve Vrouwe Gasthuis, Amsterdam, The Netherlands

Key Words

Rectum, computed tomography · Neoplasms · Rectal cancer surgery · Circumferential resection margin

Abstract

Purpose: To determine the accuracy of conventional computed tomography (CT) scan in the preoperative prediction of an involved circumferential resection margin (CRM) in primary rectal cancer. ***Methods:*** 125 patients with biopsy-proven adenocarcinoma of the rectum underwent CT of the abdomen before undergoing total mesorectal excision. Scans were scored by three observers, differing in experience. The main outcome was yes/no involvement of the CRM. Histology was taken as reference standard. ***Results:*** For the most experienced observer, observer A, sensitivity was 46.7% and specificity 92.6%. For observer B, sensitivity was 46.7% and specificity 89.5%. For the least experienced observer C, sensitivity was 43.3% and specificity 92.6%. Inter-observer variability was good between observers A and B (κ 0.648), B and C (κ 0.648), and intermediate between A and C (κ 0.542). Discrepancies occurred in a total of 34 patients; 25 had a CT scan of low technical quality, 10 an anteriorly located distal tumor. ***Conclusion:*** Conventional CT scan lacks sensitivity for a clinical use in the preoperative assessment of an involved CRM in primary rectal cancer. Modern multislice spiral CT will probably resolve some of the problems of conventional CT; however, further research is needed to establish its role.

Introduction

Successful treatment of primary rectal cancer means achieving a free circumferential resection margin (CRM). Total mesorectal excision (TME) is now the standard treatment, allowing recurrence rates below 10% [1–5]. In addition to TME, neoadjuvant treatment decreases the local recurrence rate even more to rates as low as 6% [6–15]. To assign the optimal neoadjuvant treatment strategy however, patients with rectal cancer high at risk of local recurrence need to be identified. The CRM is known to be one of the main risk factors in rectal cancer surgery [16]. A reliable prediction of the CRM by preoperative imaging is therefore important.

KARGER

Fax +41 61 306 12 34
E-Mail karger@karger.ch
www.karger.com

0257–2753/07/0251–0080$23.50/0

Accessible online at:
www.karger.com/ddi

T. Wiggers
Department of Surgery
University Medical Center Groningen, PO Box 30001
NL–9700 RB Groningen (The Netherlands)
Tel. +31 50 361 2301, Fax +31 50 361 1745, E-Mail t.wiggers@chir.umcg.nl

Recent publications have shown that MRI using phased-array coils can predict the CRM preoperatively with high accuracy [17–19].

Despite the widespread use of computed tomography (CT) in tumor staging, so far its role in the preoperative assessment of the CRM in rectal cancer staging has not been determined. In contrast to MRI, CT is more available, less expensive and less time-consuming. Furthermore, if CT would work for CRM assessment in rectal cancer patients, it would become a potential one-stop shop whole-body staging tool allowing accurate local and distant staging in one single examination.

The aim of this study is to investigate the accuracy of conventional CT for the prediction of an involved CRM in patients with primary rectal cancer.

Materials and Methods

The study was approved by the institutional review board.

Study Population

The study was performed on a retrospective basis. A cohort of patients was drawn from an existing database from the Dutch TME trial [9]. All 600 patients registered to have had a preoperative CT scan were included. All patients had a biopsy-proven, primary adenocarcinoma of the rectum, deemed primarily resectable on the basis of clinical evaluation, endoscopy and/or imaging. All patients underwent a conventional CT scan of the abdomen/pelvis before undergoing either surgery or radiotherapy. All patients underwent TME surgery performed by expert surgeons or surgeons trained by these experts to perform TME surgery. Pathologists were trained to dissect the resection specimen according to the protocol of Quirke et al. [20] and histopathological results were reviewed by a panel of supervising pathologists.

Imaging Techniques

The Dutch TME trial was a multicenter trial in which the imaging protocol was not standardized. The scans were therefore performed on different types of CT scanners and each participating hospital used its own protocol and indications for abdominal/pelvic imaging. Sections were obtained in a range of 5–15 mm with an average of 8.97 mm. All scans were made using intravenous contrast administration and a total of 81 patients had rectal contrast administered (table 1).

Table 1. Imaging techniques

Sections	Patients	IV contrast	Rectal contrast	Helical
5 mm	16	16	10	16
6 mm	3	3	0	3
7 mm	14	14	13	14
8 mm	9	9	4	9
10 mm	77	77	51	60
12 mm	2	2	0	0
15 mm	4	4	3	0
Total	125	125	81	102

Image Evaluation

In daily practice, primary rectal cancer will mostly be treated by radiotherapists and surgeons. Both these specialties will feel the need to be able to easily interpret the preoperative imaging. A member of both these specialties was therefore chosen as observer, along with a radiologist as reference observer. Images were therefore retrospectively evaluated on film by a radiologist (A), radiotherapist (B) and a surgeon (C), all acknowledged experts in the field of rectal cancer and working in different hospitals. Each observer had a different level of experience, observer A as an expert on reading both pelvic CT and MRI being the most experienced reader of pelvic and or abdominal CT scans (having read approx. 5,000 scans), observer B intermediate (having read approx. 2,000 scans) and observer C the least experienced reader (having read approx. 500 scans). All three observers assessed the scans individually and were blinded for each other's and histological results and any other patient data. None of the observers was treating physicians of the patients, and none had previous knowledge of any patient data prior to reading the images.

The scans were scored using a standardized scoring form, in which technical data were registered. The main outcome parameters were yes/no tumor involvement of the mesorectal fascia. The direction of the tumor penetration through the rectal wall was recorded as it is this direction which determines the shortest distance from the tumor to the mesorectal fascia (the CRM). In addition, the distance to the anal verge of the tumor and sites of extramesorectal growth were registered. For the prediction of the involvement, the direction of an involved fascia and the infiltration of mesorectal fat, the following confidence levels were scored: 0 = definitely not, 1 = probably not, 2 = possibly so, 3 = probably so, and 4 = definitely so.

Analysis and Statistics

The distance from the tumor to the mesorectal fascia on pathology was taken as the reference standard against which the CT findings were compared. Overall accuracy, sensitivity and specificity of the prediction of involvement of the CRM were calculated using cross-tabulation statistics. Receiver operating characteristic (ROC) analysis for the prediction of an involved mesorectal fascia were performed on the data generated by the confidence level scoring of the three observers. For each observer the accuracy of the CT for the prediction of an involved CRM was measured by calculating the area under the curve (AUC). Differences in accuracy between the observers were evaluated by a pairwise comparison of their respective areas under the ROC curve. The inter-observer agreement was measured using the linear weighted κ statistic by pairwise comparison of the accuracy of the three observers for the prediction of an involved CRM. Statistical analysis was performed using the software package SPSS® for Windows Version 11.0 (SPSS, Chicago, Ill., USA).

Table 2. Distribution of positive and negative CRM

			CRM neg	CRM pos	Total (%)
pT0	N0	M0	2	–	2 (1.6)
pT1	N0	M0	3	–	3 (2.4)
pT2	N0	M0	28	–	28 (22.4)
pT2	N1	M0	5	–	5 (4.0)
pT2	N1	M1	1	–	1 (0.8)
pT3	N0	M0	31	8	39 (31.2)
pT3	N1	M0	20	9[1]	29 (23.2)
pT3	N1	M1	3	5[2]	8 (6.4)
pT4	N0	M0	1	–	1 (0.8)
pT4	N0	M1	–	1	1 (0.8)
pT4	N1	M0	1	5	6 (4.8)
pT4	N1	M1	–	2[3]	2 (1.6)
		95 (76%)	30 (24%)		

[1] Two of these 9 patients had a positive CRM due to a positive lymph node.
[2] One of these 5 patients had a positive CRM due to a positive lymph node.
[3] One of these 2 patients had a positive CRM due to a positive lymph node.

Results

Patients

The study population consisted of 125 patients: 90 male (72%) and 35 female (28%). The age of the patients ranged between 32 and 87 with a median age of 64. The study population was a good representation of the population of the TME trial [9], in age and sex as well as in distribution of T stage.

TNM Stage

There were 2 T0 tumors, 3 T1 tumors, 34 T2 tumors, 76 T3 tumors and 10 T4 tumors. Table 2 shows the histological TNM classification of the tumors and the histological CRM assessment: free (e.g. CRM neg) or involved (CRM pos).

Prediction of Involved CRM per Observer

All three observers made 125 predictions. Thus, a total of 375 predictions were made, of which 73 were incorrect (19.5%) and 302 correct (80.5%).

Observer A was correct in 14/30 patients with positive margins and in 88/95 patients with negative margins. Observer B was correct in 14/30 patients with a positive margin and 85/95 patients with a negative margin. Observer C was correct in 13/30 patients with a positive margin and 88/95 patients with a negative margin. The sensitivity and specificity for the prediction of an involved CRM per observer are given in table 3.

Table 3. Sensitivity and specificity per observer for prediction of involved CRM

	Observer A	Observer B	Observer C
Sensitivity, %	46.7	46.7	43.3
Specificity, %	92.6	89.5	92.6

Inter-Observer Agreement

Inter-observer agreement for prediction of an involved CRM was high between observer A and observer B (κ 0.648), intermediate between observer A and observer C (κ 0.542), and high between observer B and observer C (κ 0.648).

Analysis of Predicted Involvement of CRM

If the confidence level of the prediction of each individual observer is taken into account, there is a rise in the specificity as confidence of the predictions increases for all three observers, as illustrated by the receiver operating curves in figures 1–3. This ROC analysis also shows that the AUC, and thus the overall accuracy is greatest for observer A (the most experienced reader) at 0.813 and the least for observer C (the least experienced reader) at 0.697.

Discussion

Conventional CT scan shows a low sensitivity but high specificity in the preoperative prediction of an involved CRM. An experienced reader performs better than a less experienced reader.

Based on the National Guidelines the main choice before the surgical treatment of rectal cancer is between short-course and long-course radiotherapy. The last one aiming on downsizing and downstaging. Preoperative assessment of the involved circumferential margin should primarily focus on a high sensitivity. A relatively low specificity results in some overtreatment with long-course radiotherapy and is less worse than under treatment in case of an involved margin.

Accuracy of the Prediction of an Involved CRM

Discrepancies between predicted CRM and histology occurred in 34 patients. In 25 of these 34 patients, all

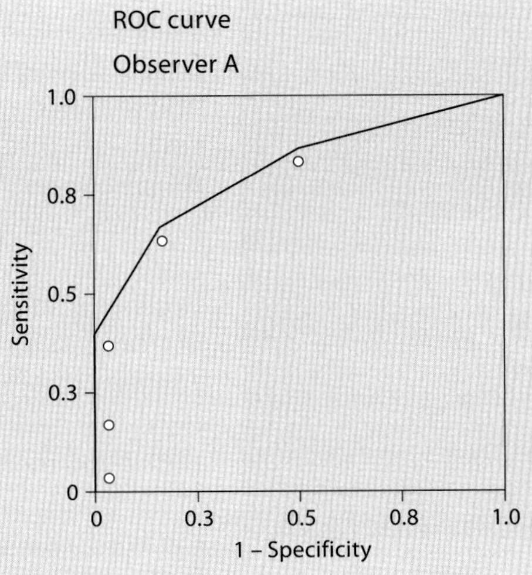

Case processing summary

Pathology confidence	Valid N (listwise)
Positive	30
Negative	94
Missing	1

Larger values of the test result variable(s) indicate stronger evidence for a positive actual state.
The positive actual state is positive.

Area under the curve

Area
0.813

Fig. 1. Receiver operating curve, cut-off points are for a positive prediction by observer A at confidence level definitely not, probably not, possibly so, probably so, and definitely so, respectively.

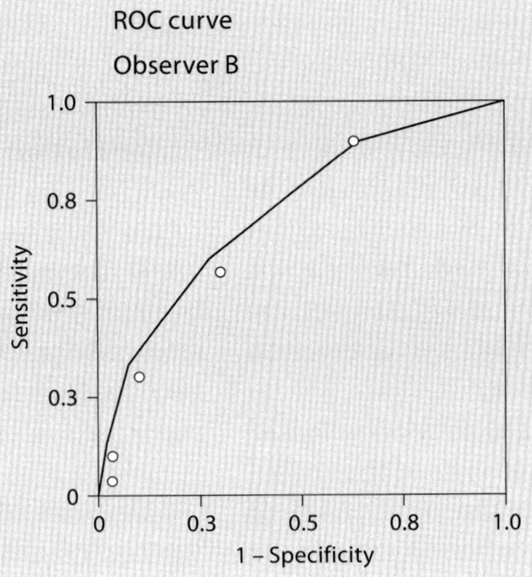

Case processing summary

Pathology confidence	Valid N (listwise)
Positive	30
Negative	95

Larger values of the test result variable(s) indicate stronger evidence for a positive actual state.
The positive actual state is positive.

Area under the curve

Area
0.723

Fig. 2. Receiver operating curve, cut-off points are for a positive prediction by observer B at confidence level definitely not, probably not, possibly so, probably so, and definitely so, respectively.

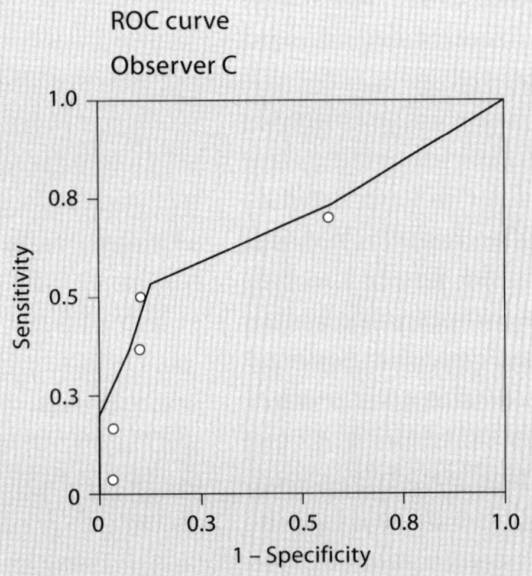

Case processing summary

Pathology confidence	Valid N (listwise)
Positive	30
Negative	94
Missing	1

Larger values of the test result variable(s) indicate stronger evidence for a positive actual state.
The positive actual state is positive.

Area under the curve

Area
0.697

Fig. 3. Receiver operating curve, cut-off points are for a positive prediction by observer C at confidence level definitely not, probably not, possibly so, probably so, and definitely so, respectively.

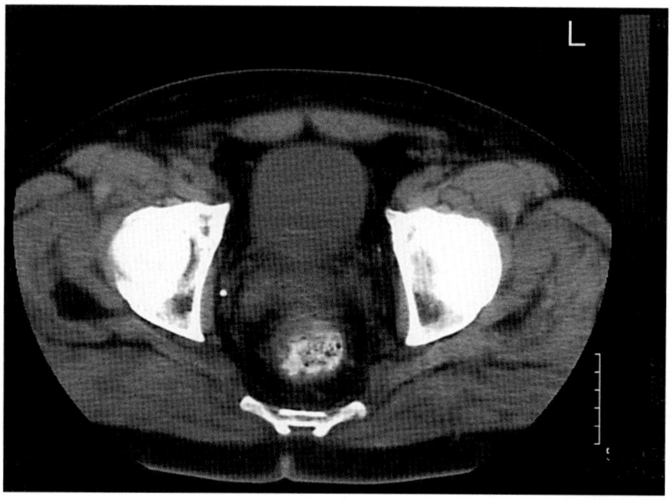

Fig. 4. Example of a CT scan in which all three observers predicted a non-involve CRM. Histology however showed an involved CRM.

MRI being superior to CT in contrast resolution and offering simultaneous imaging in different planes can better distinguish between tumor tissue and rectal wall and is expected to perform better than CT for predicting involvement of the CRM in this specific group of distal rectal cancer. Modern state-of-the-art multislice spiral CT (MSCT) however might probably do better than conventional CT, given the ability to reconstruct thinner sections and to optimally time the bolus contrast, leading not only to an improved spatial but also to an improved contrast resolution. In addition, MSCT offers reconstructions in multiple planes (multiplanar reconstruction) thus allowing an assessment of the rectal tumor in any given plane, analog to MRI. Therefore it seems justified to investigate the role of MSCT in rectal cancer staging, because if MSCT would work, it would become a potential one-stop shop whole-body staging tool allowing accurate local and distant staging in one single examination.

three observers judged the CT scan difficult to interpret due to limited spatial resolution. The main reason for the lack of sensitivity therefore seems to be of a technical nature. Most CT protocols in this study made use of thick slices (>8 mm). Therefore, the spatial resolution of the scans were too low to make any reliable predictions on margin involvement.

Most false-negatives also occurred in patients who had a distal tumor located on the anterior side of the mesorectum with a threatened margin anteriorly. In these false-negative cases the margins were often involved only by subtle tumor stranding. Because of the inherent lack of contrast resolution of CT and the insufficient spatial resolution of conventional CT techniques in this study, these tumor strands were not visualized on the CT and therefore missed by all observers (fig. 4).

Second, many disagreements between CT and histology occurred on where the tumor exactly penetrates the bowel wall. The exact location of the site of tumor penetration is essential when the site of the closest CRM has to be anticipated, because it is at this site where the mesorectal fascia should be scrutinized for any possible invasion by tumor stranding. Again, the very low contrast resolution of conventional CT prevents clear distinction between the bowel wall and tumor tissue, making it very difficult to predict the site of bowel wall penetration, resulting in misinterpretations of the site of margin involvement.

Conclusion

Conventional CT scan lacks sensitivity for a clinical use in the preoperative assessment of an involved CRM in primary rectal cancer. Modern MSCT will probably resolve some of the problems of conventional CT; however, further research is needed to establish its role.

References

1 Heald RJ, Husband EM, Ryall RDH: The mesorectum in rectal surgery: The clue to pelvic recurrence? Br J Surg 1982;69:613–606.
2 Havenga K, Enker WE, Norstein J, Moriya Y, Heald RJ, van Houwelingen HC, et al: Improved survival and local control after mesorectal excision or D3 lymphadenectomy in the treatment of primary rectal cancer: an international analysis of 1,411 patients. Eur J Surg Oncol 1999;25:368–374.
3 MacFarlane JK, Ryall RDH, Heald RJ: Mesorectal excision for rectal cancer. Lancet 1993; 341:457–460.
4 Enker WE, Thaler HT, Cranor ML, Polyak T: Total mesorectal excision in the operative treatment of carcinoma of the rectum. J Am Coll Surg 1995;181:335–346.
5 Aitken RJ: Mesorectal excision for rectal cancer. Br J Surg 1996;83:214–216.
6 Colorectal Cancer Collaborative Group: Adjuvant radiotherapy for rectal cancer: a systematic overview of 8,507 patients from 22 randomised trials. Lancet 2001;358:1291–1303.
7 Investigators Swedish Rectal Cancer Trial: Improved survival with preoperative radiotherapy in resectable rectal cancer. N Engl J Med 1997;336:980–987.
8 Marijnen CAM, Glimelius B: The role of radiotherapy in rectal cancer. Eur J Cancer 2002;38:943–952.
9 Kapiteijn E, Marijnen CAM, Nagtegaal ID, Putter H, Steup W, Wiggers T, et al: Preoperative radiotherapy combined with total mesorectal excision for resectable rectal cancer. N Engl J Med 2001;345:638–646.
10 Marijnen CAM, Nagtegaal ID, Kapiteijn E, Klein-Kranenberg E, Noorddijk EM, van Krieken HJM, et al: Radiotherapy does not compensate for positive resection margins in rectal cancer patients. Radiotherapy in rectal cancer. Thesis. ISBN 9090156356:91–103.
11 Marijnen CAM, Nagtegaal ID, Klein-Kranenbarg E, Hermans J, van de Velde CJ, Leer JW, et al: No downstaging after short-term pre-operative radiotherapy in rectal cancer patients. J Clin Oncol 2001;19:1976–1984.
12 Glimelius B, Isacson U: Preoperative radiotherapy for rectal cancer – is 5 × 5 Gy a good or a bad schedule? Acta Oncol 2001;40:958–967.
13 Steele RJ, Sebag-Montefiore D: Adjuvant radiotherapy for rectal cancer. Br J Surg 1999; 86:1233–1234.
14 Medical Research Council Working Party: Randomised trial of surgery alone versus surgery followed by radiotherapy for mobile cancer of the rectum. Lancet 1996;348:1610–1614.
15 Krook JE, Moertel CG, Gunderson LL, Wieanand HS, Collins RT, Beart RW, et al: Effective surgical adjuvant therapy for high-risk rectal carcinoma. N Engl J Med 1991; 324:709–715.
16 Nagtegaal ID, Marijnen CA, Kranenbarg EK, van de Velde CJ, van Krieken JH: Circumferential margin involvement is still an important predictor of local recurrence in rectal carcinoma: not one millimeter but two millimeters is the limit. Am J Surg Pathol 2002;26:350–357.
17 Beets Tan RGH, Beets GJ, Vliegen RFA, Kessels AG, Van Boven H, De Bruine A, et al: Accuracy of MRI in prediction of tumor free resection margin in rectal cancer surgery. Lancet 2001;357:497–504.
18 Brown G, Richards CJ, Newcombe RG, Dallimore NS, Radcliffe AG, Carey DP, et al: Rectal carcinoma: thin section MR imaging for staging in 28 patients. Radiology 1999: 221;215–229.
19 Lahaye MJ, Engelen SM, Nelemans PJ, Beets GL, van de Velde CJ, van Engelshoven JM, et al: Imaging for predicting the risk factors – the circumferential resection margin and nodal disease – of local recurrence in rectal cancer: a meta-analysis. Semin Ultrasound CT MR 2005;26:259–268.
20 Quirke P, Durdey P, Dixon MF, Williams NS: Local recurrence of rectal adenocarcinoma due to inadequate surgical resection. Histopathological study of lateral tumour spread and surgical excision Lancet 1986;ii:996–999.

Original Article

Digestive Diseases

Dig Dis 2007;25:86–93
DOI: 10.1159/000099175

Detection of Colorectal Cancer Hepatic Metastases with Contrast-Enhanced Ultrasound: Comparison with Conventional B-Mode Ultrasound

S.D. Yarmenitis A. Karantanas A. Bakantaki Y. Papantoniou N. Gourtsoyiannis

Department of Radiology, University of Crete, Faculty of Medicine, Heraklion, Greece

Key Words
Colorectal cancer/imaging · Liver neoplasms/ultrasonography · Contrast media · Metastatic disease/diagnosis

Abstract
The aim of this study was to assess whether contrast-enhanced ultrasound (CE-US) could provide improved diagnostic information in detecting liver metastases from colorectal cancer as compared to B-mode non-enhanced ultrasound (B-US). 32 patients (M/F 23/9, age range 48–82 years, mean 58.2 years) under chemotherapy for colorectal cancer were examined with B-US and CE-US using a second-generation ultrasound contrast agent and a dedicated protocol for contrast detection. The presence of focal liver lesions along with the number, size, pre- and post-contrast sonographic features were recorded digitally. Lesion conspicuity with a three-grade scoring scale was performed on both techniques and contrast intensity measurements were calculated for each focal lesion. CE-US detected 17% more metastases in patient-by-patient and lesion-by-lesion analysis. A statistically significant difference was found between the scoring mean values with regard to conspicuity of the lesions. Accurate characterization of the liver lesions was achievable only with contrast-enhanced technique. A quantitative contrast intensity measurement method confirmed the invariably washing-out vascular pattern in all metastases at sinusoidal-parenchymal liver phase. In conclusion, CE-US is superior to B-US and provides an effective tool in the investigation of colorectal cancer liver metastases.

Introduction

The early detection and precise characterization of liver metastases from colorectal carcinoma has become a crucial issue in treatment planning and is also considered to be important for improved therapeutic outcomes. In most of colorectal cancer patients, conventional B-mode non-enhanced ultrasound (B-US) is the first-line imaging modality for detecting liver metastases. However, US in the detection of focal liver lesions presents a sensitivity ranging from 40 to 80% according to the diameter of lesions and to the experience of the sonologist [1, 2].

The introduction of ultrasound contrast agents and the advances in ultrasound apparatuses that are now able to detect these agents in real time have improved the overall accuracy of US in the characterization of focal liver lesions [3, 4], in liver metastases detection [5–10] and in monitoring the effect of therapy in liver metastases [11].

KARGER

Fax +41 61 306 12 34
E-Mail karger@karger.ch
www.karger.com

0257–2753/07/0251–0086$23.50/0

Accessible online at:
www.karger.com/ddi

A. Karantanas, MD, PhD
Department of Radiology, University Hospital
GR–711 10 Stavrakia/Heraklion (Greece)
Tel. +30 2810 392 541, Fax +30 2810 542 095
E-Mail apolsen@yahoo.com or karantanas@med.uoc.gr

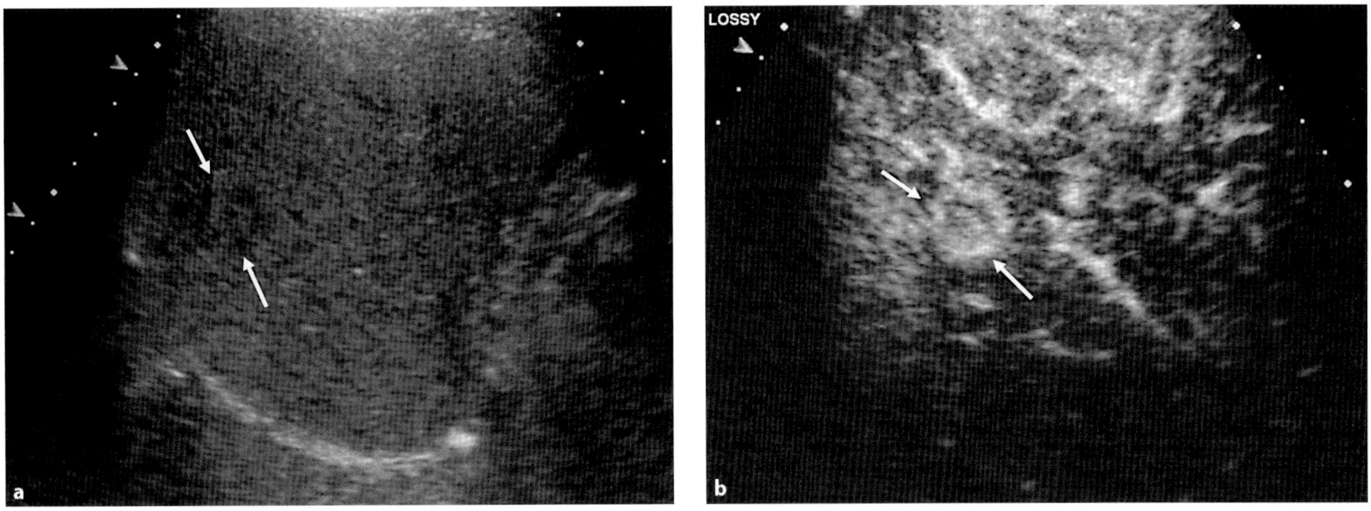

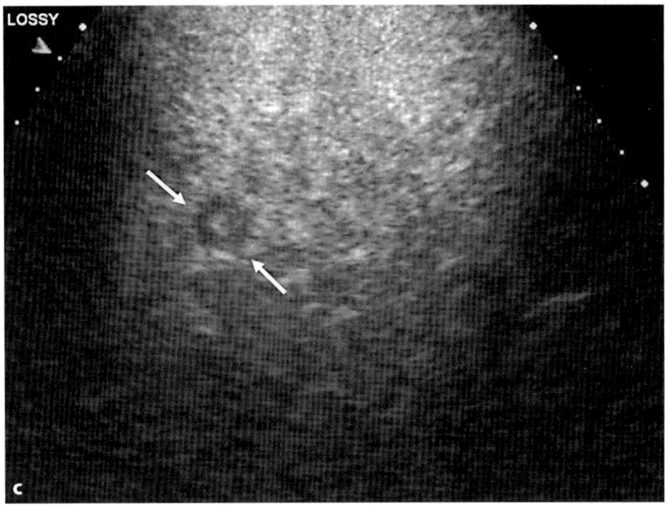

Fig. 1. A 55-year-old male patient with history of rectal carcinoma under chemotherapy and regular imaging follow-up. **a** The 2-year non-enhanced B-US discloses a target-like liver metastatic lesion with isoechoic center and hypoechoic margin (arrows). **b** CE-US at post-injection arterial liver phase shows the hypervascular characteristics of the lesion (arrows). **c** In the sinusoidal-parenchymal liver phase CE-US, there is contrast agent washout and the lesion appears hypovascular against the surrounding liver parenchyma (arrows).

A recent study [12] compared contrast-enhanced ultrasound (CE-US) with B-US and contrast-enhanced spiral CT in metastatic, of any primary cancer, disease of the liver. CE-US was found to have an 83% sensitivity, 84% specificity and a high accuracy as shown by a 0.929 ROC under the curve analysis.

Since the introduction of CE-US, all published data on the investigation of hepatic metastatic disease refer to hepatic metastases secondary to any primary. To our knowledge, there are no reports in the English literature that assess the performance of this new method exclusively on the colorectal cancer liver metastases.

Our purpose in this study was to evaluate whether the detection and characterization of liver metastases from colorectal carcinoma can be improved by using CE-US, as compared with non-enhanced B-US.

Materials and Methods

Over a period of 1 year, 32 consecutive patients (23 males and 9 females, age range 48–82 years, mean age 58.2 years) under chemotherapy for a diagnosed colorectal carcinoma, were included in this study. An overall informed consent for diagnostic and therapeutic procedures, including the pre- and post-contrast ultrasound studies of the liver, was promptly provided to the referring physicians. Approval from the ethics committee of our institution was not needed since CE-US of the liver is among the labeled indications of the specific US contrast agent that was used in this study.

All patients were examined with a Siemens, Acuson Sequoia 512 (Signature II Version 8) ultrasound unit equipped with a 4C1, 2–4-MHz curved array abdominal transducer. A non-enhanced B-US investigation preceded all CE-US studies. Tissue harmonic and spatial compounding software were used as a standard preset for the B-US scans in order to reduce noise and speckle artifacts in an effort to increase baseline lesion conspicuity. The contrast-

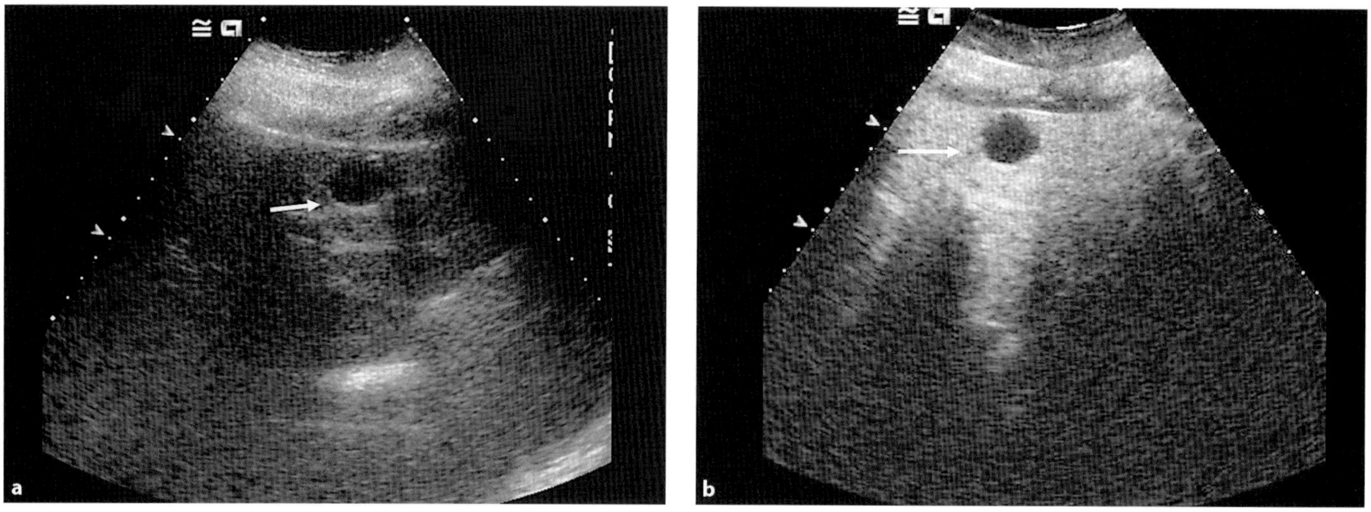

Fig. 2. A parenchymal liver cyst at non-enhanced B-US (**a**) and CE-US (**b**) appears totally anechoic with sharp borders and posterior echo enhancement (arrow).

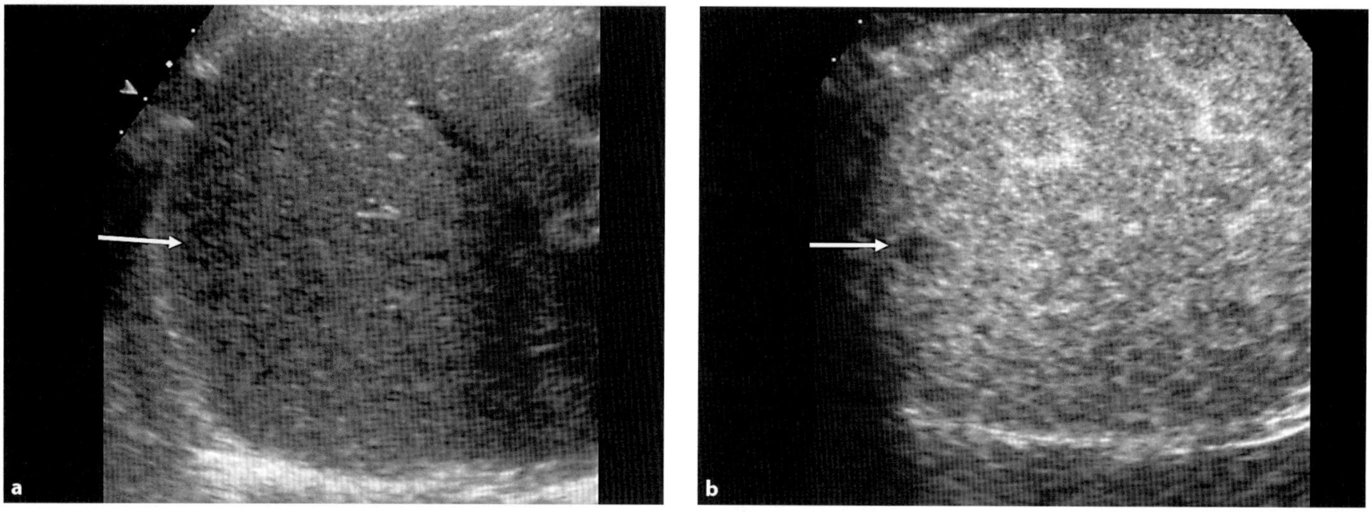

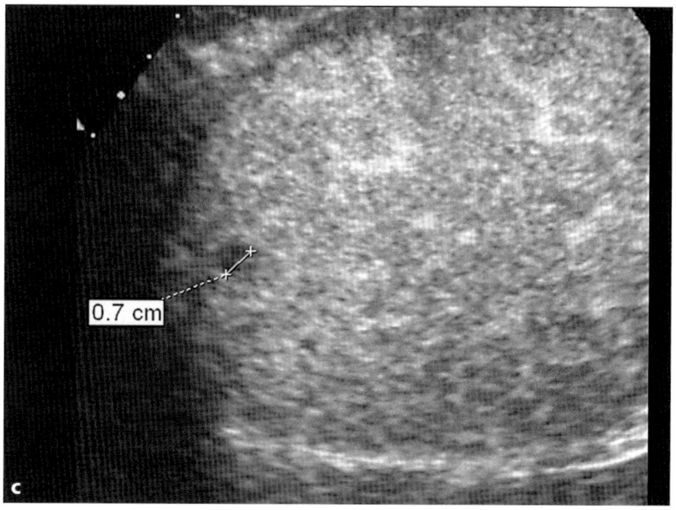

Fig. 3. Patient with left colon carcinoma, operated 3 years prior to imaging. **a** The non-enhanced B-US of right liver lobe shows a suspected focal liver lesion (arrow) with extremely poor conspicuity and lack of tissue reflectivity differentiation. CE-US (**b**) reveals a subcentimeter (**c**) hypovascularized colorectal cancer metastasis (arrow). Detection and characterization was impossible with baseline US.

specific scan protocol was based on the Contrast Pulse Sequencing (CPS) software for low mechanical index contrast detection.

SonoVue Bracco Sulfur hexafluoride (SF6) microbubbles were used as ultrasound contrast agent at a standard intravenous dose of 2.4 ml. A supplementary dose of 2.4 ml was occasionally administered to ascertain diagnostic information in some cases. A third dose was never required. The perfusion process was evaluated in real time, utilizing CPS mode ability to interchange between contrast only, mixed or B-mode only imaging. All studies were recorded with the use of dedicated software in digital video sequences lasting for 3 min at least. Off-line workstation reading of the recorded ultrasound examinations followed thereafter by two on-site radiologists (S.D.Y. with 20 and 6 years of ultrasound and contrast studies experience, and A.B. with 15 and 3 years experience respectively).

From the review of the digital recordings, each case was assessed for the presence or not of focal liver lesions. Thereafter the lesion number, size and characteristic patterns on B-US and on CE-US were recorded and a three-grade lesion conspicuity score was applied on both techniques as follows: grade 3 for lesions that showed optimum conspicuity, grade 2 for suboptimal conspicuity and grade 1 for poor or no conspicuity at all. The grading was done in a side-by-side fashion and final scoring decision was reported by consensus. Statistical analysis was performed with Mann-Whitney test for the lesion conspicuity grading. The CE-US features for diagnosing a metastasis were those of a hyper- or hypoenhancing lesion at 15–20 s post-contrast injection followed by a clear washout of the contrast agent at 60–90 s post-injection resulting in a hypovascular focus against hyperenhanced neighboring liver parenchyma (fig. 1) [13].

Hemangiomas were diagnosed when a lesion showed either gradual slow peripheral centripetal enhancement or rapid initial overall enhancement but with continuous persistent hyperenhancement throughout the study.

Contrast intensity measurement was performed for each detected lesion using the Merge Efilm Workstation Version 1.8 software by defining regions of interest (ROI). Arbitrary intensity values were taken from each ROI at 20 and 60 s post-contrast injection.

The final diagnosis of those lesions considered as metastatic was established with biopsy or multimodality imaging assessment with characteristic findings on contrast-enhanced CT or MR imaging including progressive enlargement or subsequent reduction in size following chemotherapy. Dynamic contrast-enhanced CT or MR imaging findings reported as showing diagnostic features of hemangioma with no change at follow-up of longer than 1 year.

Table 1. Number of detected lesions and corresponding lesion conspicuity score in each one of the US techniques (non-marked cases correspond to metastatic lesions cases)

Patients' initials	Number of lesions, non-enhanced US	Number of lesions CE-US	Conspicuity score non-enhanced US mean: 2.23$^+$	Conspicuity score, CE-US mean: 2.82$^+$
HS**	1	1	3	3
PI	2	2	2	3
MS	0	2	1	3
ME**	3	4	3	3
MM*	0	0		
KE	>5	>10	2	3
KA*	0	0		
ZG	0	1	1	3
BZ*	0	0		
PN	1	2	1	2
MG*	0	0		
BG*	0	0		
BM*	0	0		
SK*	0	0		
ZN*	0	0		
PK**	2	2	2	2
KM*	0	0		
KH**	2	2	3	3
TK[a]	0	1	1	3
PE[a, **]	2	2	2	3
KF*	0	0		
TN	>10	>10	3	3
HD	1	1	3	3
KA*	0	0	1	1[b]
MS	1	1	3	3
MM*	0	0	3	3
GK[a]	1	1	2	3
KK	3	3	3	3
HN*	0	0	3	3
GH	0	2	1	3
IV	3	3	3	3
LE[c]	3	3	3	3

Conspicuity score: 1 = poor; 2 = suboptimal; 3 = optimal lesion conspicuity.

* No lesions found. ** Parenchymal cysts.

[a] Hemangioma. [b] Fatty liver. [c] Calcified metastases (primary mucinous adenocarcinoma). $^+$ $p = 0.001$: statistical significance of the difference of conspicuity score mean values, between the non-enhanced and contrast-enhanced ultrasound.

Results

No lesions were found in 13 patients at both B-US and CE-US. In 2 of these individuals, CE-CT revealed 1 and 2 subcentimeter lesions respectively. One of these turned out to be a metastasis in a subsequent follow-up CT scan, whereas the others remained unchanged. It was not feasible to define with contrast-enhanced helical CT whether these two lesions were tiny cysts or hemangiomas.

Nineteen individuals showed focal lesions. Both ultrasound techniques revealed ten parenchymal cysts in 5 patients ranging from 0.6 to 3.6 cm (fig. 2). Two of them were subcentimeter lesions (0.6 and 0.7 cm). Two hyperechoic solitary hemangiomas 1.2 and 2.7 cm were detected by both US modes in 2 patients. A third hypoechoic 1-cm lesion in another patient, in B-US, turned out to be

Table 2. Size and pre- and post-contrast echographic patterns of lesions

Initials	Size, cm	Pattern non-enhanced US	Pattern CE-US (arterial-sinusoidal phases)
HS	0.6	cyst	cyst
PI	2	hypoechoic with isoechoic center	hypervascular with persistent rim – hypovascular
	2.7	hypoechoic with isoechoic center	hypervascular with persistent rim – hypovascular
MS	1.2	isoechoic	hypovascular-hypovascular
	0.7	isoechoic	hypovascular-hypovascular
ME	3.6	cyst	cyst
	2.2	cyst	cyst
	3.1	cyst	cyst
	1	cyst	cyst
KE	5 mets	hypoechoic	hypovascular-hypovascular
ZG	2.4	isoechoic	hypovascular-hypovascular
PN	4	hypoechoic	hypovascular-hypovascular
	1.2	isoechoic	hypovascular-hypovascular
PK	1.4	cyst	cyst
	1	cyst	cyst
KH	1.5	cyst	cyst
	1.4	cyst	cyst
TK*	1	hypoechoic	hypovascular-isovascular
PE*	1.2	hyperechoic	hypervascular-hypervascular
	1	cyst	cyst
TN	numerous mets	hypoechoic and hyperechoic	Hypovascular-hypovascular
HD	1.2	hypoechoic	hypovascular-hypovascular
MS	1.8	hypoechoic with isoechoic center	hypervascular with persistent rim – hypovascular
GK*	hemangioma 2.7	hyperechoic	hypervascular-hypervascular
KK	2.4	hypoechoic with isoechoic center	hypovascular-hypovascular
	2	hypoechoic with isoechoic center	hypovascular-hypovascular
	2	hypoechoic with isoechoic center	hypovascular-hypovascular
GH	1	isoechoic	hypovascular-hypovascular
	1.8	isoechoic	hypovascular-hypovascular
IV	3.7	hypoechoic with isoechoic center	hypervascular with persistent rim – hypovascular
	3.4	hypoechoic with isoechoic center	hypervascular with persistent rim – hypovascular
	3	hypoechoic with isoechoic center	hypervascular with persistent rim – hypovascular
LE	6	hypoechoic with isoechoic center calcifications	hypervascular with persistent rim – hypovascular
	3	hypoechoic with isoechoic center calcifications	hypervascular with persistent rim – hypovascular
	3	hypoechoic with isoechoic center calcifications	hypervascular with persistent rim – hypovascular

* Hemangioma.

a hemangioma on CE-US. One cyst and one hemangioma coexisted in 1 patient.

A total of 12 (37.5%) patients were diagnosed as having hepatic metastases. Eleven of them had 1–5 lesions and 1 presented with diffuse metastatic disease. Ten patients (83%) were found to have metastases with both US techniques, whereas 2 (17%) were diagnosed only with CE-US. Of these 2 individuals, 1 had a solitary isoechoic metastasis of 2.4 cm and the other had two isoechoic metastases of 0.7 and 1.2 cm (fig. 3).

On a lesion-by-lesion basis and after excluding 1 patient with diffuse disease, a total of 32 metastatic foci (59%) were localized by both US techniques, whereas 9 metastatic foci (17%) were detected only with CE-US (tables 1, 2).

Various patterns of echogenicity were found in the baseline non-enhanced US for the metastatic foci (ill-defined isoechoic n = 6, hypoechoic n = 4, and target-like hypoechoic with isoechoic center n = 12). On CE-US all metastatic lesions were invariably hypovascular at the parenchymal-sinusoidal phase at 40–90 s post-contrast injection. However, nine lesions showed a hypervascular activity during the arterial phase, 15–25 s post-contrast injection, and all were of the target-like 'hypoechoic with

Table 3. Contrast intensity measurements of metastatic foci and hemangiomas at arterial and sinusoidal liver phases

Initials	Intensity values arterial phase	Intensity values sinusoidal-parenchymal phase
PI	98.5	77.5
	100	83.2
MS	77.7	68.9
	**	87
ZG	97.4	72.6
PN	93.1	60.4
	115.2	57.3
TK*	31.6	57.4
PE*	153.2	163.5
HD	57	42
MS	117.6	65.4
GK*	65.8	87.3
KK	109.3	72.2
	99.3	73
	98	67.5
GH	70	58
	74	63
IV	97.1	67.5
	92	68
	95.6	60.7
LE	87	58
	91.6	63.4
	86.7	60.8

Intensity values are arbitrary measurements of contrast intensity calculated by Merge Efilm Workstation Version 1.8 by defining regions of interest (ROI) at the specific lesions at 20 and 60 s post-injection.

* Hemangioma. ** Arterial phase missing.

isoechoic center' pattern at the baseline US. The rest of the lesions were of the hypovascular type during the arterial phase. It is interesting that this hypovascularity at the arterial phase was presented by all as the ill-defined 'isoechoic' type of metastases that were not detectable at the baseline non-enhanced US (table 2).

The contrast intensity calculations yielded overlapping values for each individual lesion and for each hepatic vascular phase, but on the other hand, all metastatic lesions showed an invariable decrease of their individual intensity values at the sinusoidal-parenchymal liver phase as compared to the corresponding values recorded at the arterial phase. In contrast to this, all three hemangiomas showed a constant increase of the contrast intensity at the sinusoidal-parenchymal liver phase (table 3, fig. 4).

The three-grade scoring (table 1) of the conspicuity of focal lesions for each one of the US techniques yielded a mean value of 2.23 for the non-enhanced US and 2.82 for the CE-US. The difference of the two means was found to be statistically significant ($p < 0.003$).

Discussion

Although several US characteristics in focal liver lesions may be related to malignancy and specifically to metastatic disease, considerable overlapping with benign lesion patterns may exist [14]. In addition, the echotexture of both liver metastases and liver parenchyma may be considerably influenced during chemotherapy resulting thus in B-mode US images that are extremely difficult to interpret. The present study shows that CE-US succeeded to diagnose colorectal liver metastases in 17% more patients and also 17% more metastases on a per-lesion basis as compared to the B-US. In the same context, the significant scoring differences regarding lesion conspicuity between B-US and CE-US underline the added value from the latter in increasing the diagnostic confidence. Among the 22 patients with focal liver lesions, the conspicuity score for CE-US was reduced (to suboptimal score 2) in only 2 patients who showed limited cooperation and presented with lesions at anatomically difficult areas. One other examinee was assigned with a score of 1 in both B-US and CE-US due to heavy hepatic steatosis. The MR imaging study of this particular patient was negative for focal liver lesions. Our results are in accordance with the guidelines of the European Federation of the Societies of Ultrasound in Medicine and Biology (EFSUMB) for the use of CE-US in the follow-up of oncological patients who have liver metastases.

In the present study, a lower rate (17%) of improved liver metastasis detection was found as opposed to the 46% reported by Quaia et al. [12]. This difference might be explained by the fact that in the study by Quaia et al., the population under study was mixed including patients suffering from various malignancies and many were imaged before chemotherapy. In the present study all examinees were follow-up colorectal cancer cases at various stages of their chemotherapy regimens. Thus the possibility of a significant remission of preexisting liver metastases should be taken seriously under consideration.

Nonetheless, apart from the issue of lesion detection, CE-US was the technique that yielded the possibility to characterize all detected hepatic lesions with certainty, a task that would have been difficult to be accomplished by

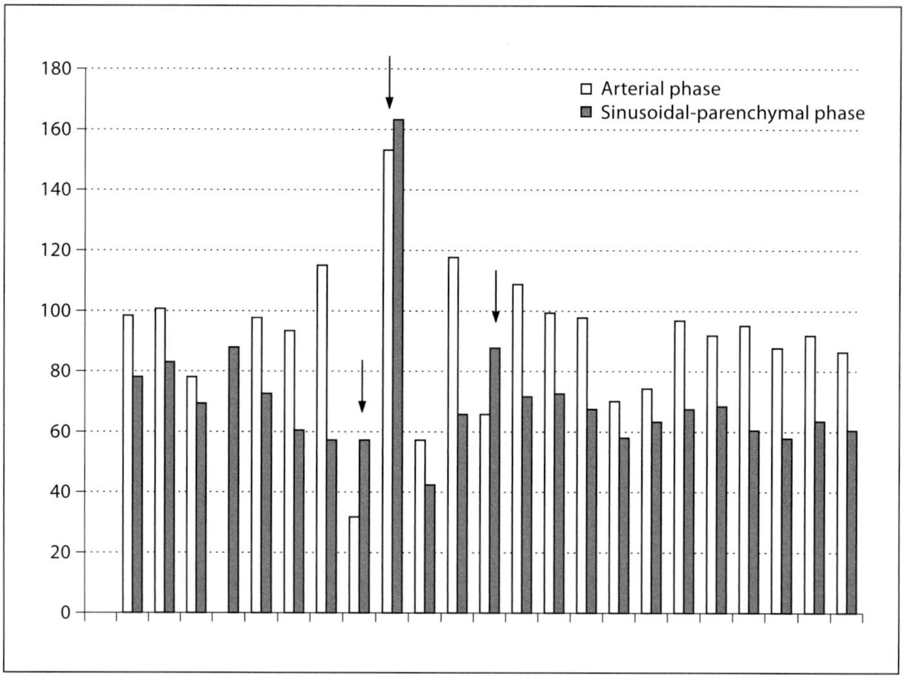

Fig. 4. A bar graph of contrast intensity values of the liver metastatic lesions and hemangiomas (arrows). Although individual values are overlapping, all metastases show clear reduction of intensity values at sinusoidal-parenchymal liver phase compared to those at the arterial phase. In contrast to this, all hemangiomas show increased values at sinusoidal-parenchymal liver phase.

B-US or without the assistance of CT or MR scans. In the present study we have also tried to introduce a quantitative technique in order to enhance the success of focal lesion identification. So far, the attempts to characterize focal liver lesions and hence hepatic metastasis with CE-US rely on a subjective qualitative comparison of the contrast enhancement of lesions against that of the surrounding liver parenchyma [4–10]. By applying direct intensity measurements at specific ROI at the individual focal lesions, we have shown that the expected contrast washout is measurable not only on the hypervascular metastases but also on the colorectal metastases with a reduced arterial supply. In a similar fashion, the hemangiomas yielded a clearly detectable increase of enhancement against time.

The observation that the isoechoic ill-defined metastases in our study population were all hypovascularized during the arterial phase poses the issue that a chemotherapy-induced altered angiogenesis combined with altered echogenicity might exist. It must be pointed out that the well-defined hypoechoic lesions in this study were also hypovascularized at the arterial phase while the target-like hypoechoic with isoechoic center lesions showed predominantly hypervascular arterial phase patterns. Prospective studies with long-term imaging follow-up are needed to clarify the previous observations.

The relatively small study population and the predominance of male patients was the probable reason that we did not detect more rare focal lesions such as focal nodular hyperplasias and hepatic adenomas.

The fact that both observers in this paper were inevitably aware of the existing primary colorectal neoplasia poses a strong potential bias towards the final diagnosis. For this reason a blinded reading of the video recordings by off-site readers should have been the appropriate choice to minimize such a possibility. However, in the present study, the exposure of all the examined individuals to a chemotherapeutic regimen provides a degree of added difficulty at the level of B-US that may have restricted this bias to some extent. Moreover, the inclusion of all examinees in a single group without a reference to preexisting liver lesions or duration of treatment, although a possible limitation as denoted below, provided a further establishment of a 'blinded' approach.

A number of limitations exist in the present study. First, due to the relatively small group of the examined individuals, we did not correlate the pre- and post-contrast echographic patterns of the liver lesions with the histologic type of the colorectal tumor, the site and stage of the primary lesion, the duration of the disease and the type and duration of the chemotherapeutic treatment. Second, we did not perform a CE-US follow-up study to define its capability to illustrate the possible serial alterations of the patterns of hepatic metastases throughout the treatment. Third, a direct correlation with CE-CT or MR was not feasible since at this point the study was only designed to compare the B-US with CE-US.

In conclusion, the present study has shown that CE-US is able to depict and characterize the colorectal cancer liver metastases with increased rates. Especially in the difficult field of altered liver echogenicity due to chemotherapy side effects, several inconsistencies that appear with non-enhanced baseline US may be solved efficiently. Quantification of the degree of enhancement adds confidence on the characterization of the metastatic lesions from colorectal cancer. Finally, the observation that the isoechoic ill-defined metastases in our study population were all hypovascularized during arterial phase has to be viewed with larger studies.

References

1 Cosgrove DO, Bolondi L: Malignant liver disease; in Cosgrove D, Meire H, Dewbury K (eds): Abdominal and General Ultrasound. Edinburgh, Churchill Livingstone, 1993, pp 271–293.

2 Wernecke K, Rummeny E, Bongartz G, et al: Detection of hepatic masses in patients with carcinoma: comparative sensitivities of sonography, CT and MR imaging. AJR Am J Roentgenol 1991;157:731–739.

3 Bleuzen A, Tranquart F: Incidental liver lesions: diagnostic value of cadence contrast pulse sequencing and SonoVue. Eur Radiol 2004;14(suppl 8):P53–P62.

4 Quaia E, Calliada F, Bertolotto M, et al: Characterization of focal liver lesions by contrast-specific US modes and a sulfur hexafluoride-filled microbubble contrast agent: diagnostic performance and confidence. Radiology 2004;232:420–430.

5 Blomley MJ, Albrecht TA, Cosgrove DO, et al: Improved detection of liver metastases with stimulated acoustic emission in late phase of enhancement with the US contrast agent SH U 508: early experience. Radiology 1999;210:409–416.

6 Harvey CJ, Blomley MJ, Eckersley RJ, et al: Hepatic malignancies: improved detection with pulse inversion US in late phase of enhancement with SH U 508 A – early experience. Radiology 2000;216:903–908.

7 Quaia E, Bertolotto M, Forgács B, et al: Detection of liver metastases by pulse inversion harmonic imaging during levovist late phase: comparison to conventional ultrasound and helical CT in 160 patients. Eur Radiol 2003; 13:475–483.

8 Albrecht T, Blomley MJK, Burns PN, et al: Improved detection of hepatic metastases with pulse-inversion US during the liver-specific phase of SHU 508A: multicenter study. Radiology 2003;227:361–370.

9 Oldenburg A, Hohmann J, Foert E, et al: Detection of hepatic metastases with low MI real time contrast-enhanced sonography and SonoVue. Ultraschall Med 2005;26:277–284.

10 Whittingham T: Contrast-specific imaging techniques: technical perspective; in Quaia E (ed): Contrast Media in Ultrasonography: Basic Principles and Clinical Applications. Berlin, Springer, 2005, pp 43–70.

11 Krix M, Plathow C, Essig M, et al: Monitoring of liver metastases after stereotactic radiotherapy using low-MI contrast-enhanced ultrasound – initial results. Eur Radiol 2005; 15:677–684.

12 Quaia E, D'Onofrio M, Palumbo A, et al: Comparison of contrast-enhanced ultrasonography versus baseline ultrasound and contrast-enhanced computed tomography in metastatic disease of the liver: diagnostic performance and confidence. Eur Radiol DOI 2006;10.1007/s00330-006-0192-7.

13 Hohmann J, Albrecht T, Hoffmann CW, et al: Ultrasonographic detection of focal liver lesions: increased sensitivity and specificity with microbubble contrast agents. Eur J Radiol 2003;46:147–159.

14 Harvey CJ, Albrecht T: Ultrasound of focal liver lesions. Eur Radiol 2001;11:1578–1593.

Original Article

Digestive Diseases

Dig Dis 2007;25:94–99
DOI: 10.1159/000099176

Lymph Node Clearance after Total Mesorectal Excision for Rectal Cancer: Laparoscopic versus Open Approach

George Pechlivanides[a] Nikolaos Gouvas[b] John Tsiaoussis[c] Anastasios Tzortzinis[d] Maria Tzardi[b] M. Moutafidis[a] Christos Dervenis[e] Evaghelos Xynos[b]

[a]First Department of General Surgery, Athens Naval Hospital, [b]Medical School, University of Crete, [c]Department of Surgery, 'Metropolitan Hospital', [d]Department of General Surgery, Naval Hospital of Crete, and [e]First Department of General Surgery, 'Agia Olga' Hospital of Athens, Greece

Key Words

Laparoscopy · Rectal cancer · Total mesorectal excision · Lymph node harvesting · Lymph node clearance

Abstract

Background: Laparoscopic resection of the rectum is still under scrutiny for its adequacy of oncological clearance. ***Aim:*** To assess lymph node yield after laparoscopic total mesorectal excision (TME) for rectal cancer as compared to the open approach. ***Methods:*** 74 patients with middle and low rectal cancer were prospectively randomized in two groups. Group A included 39 patients who had an open TME (35 with low anterior resection of the rectum (LARR) and 4 with abdominoperineal resection of the rectum (APR)). In group B, there were 34 patients who had a laparoscopic TME (27 with LARR and 7 with APR). 10 of the LARR patients in group A and 14 of the LARR patients in group B had a defunctioning ileostomy. All operations were performed by one surgeon or under his supervision. ***Results:*** Gender and age distribution were similar for both groups (group A: 23 males; mean age 69 (41–85); group B: 20 males; mean age 72 (31–84)). The mean distance of the tumor from the dentate line was 7.6 cm (1–12 cm) for group A and 6.1 cm (1–12 cm) for group B. Anastomosis was formed at a mean distance of 5.5 cm (1.5–8.5 cm) from the dentate line in group A and 3.5 cm (1–4.5 cm) in group B. At histology, in group A there were 5 T4 tumors, 9 T3, 10 T3+ (<1 mm distance from the circumferential resection margin), 13 T2 and 2 T1. In group B, there were 3 T4 tumors, 14 T3, 8 T3+, 7 T2 and 2 T1. Differences between groups were not significant. The mean number of lymph nodes retrieved in group A specimens was 19.2 (5–45) and in group B 19.2 (8–41) ($p = 0.2$). In group A, 3.9 (1–9) regional, 13.9 (3–34) intermediate and 1.5 (1–3) apical lymph nodes were retrieved. The respective values in group B were 3.7 (3–7), 14.4 (4–33) and 1.3 (1–3). Differences between groups were not significant. Also, the incidence of lymph node involvement by the tumor was not significantly different between groups (group A: 23; group B: 19). ***Conclusions:*** Laparoscopic resection of the rectum can achieve similar lymph node clearance to the open approach. Also, distribution of the lymph nodes along the resected specimens is similar between the two approaches.

KARGER

Fax +41 61 306 12 34
E-Mail karger@karger.ch
www.karger.com

0257–2753/07/0251–0094$23.50/0

Accessible online at:
www.karger.com/ddi

Evaghelos Xynos
19, Michelidaki Street
GR–712 02 Heraklion (Greece)
Tel. +30 2810 280 002, Fax +30 2810 280 009
E-Mail exynos@med.uoc.gr

Introduction

Standardization of mesorectal excision for rectal cancer as proposed by Heald et al. [1] undoubtedly resulted in lower local recurrence [2] and longer survival [3] rates as compared to conventional resection of the rectum. To date, there is evidence that laparoscopy for colorectal cancer offers the chance for a meticulous and easy dissection of the mesocolon and mesorectum under direct vision, in contrast to the 'touch-guided' open approach, particularly applied when dealing with the rectum. According to two recent meta-analyses [4, 5], there is enough evidence that laparoscopic surgery can achieve oncological clearance equal to the open approach for rectal cancer. The evidence presented is not strong, mostly because it is based on randomized trials with rather small number of patients included [6–8], one multicentric trial [9] and several cohort studies [10–25]. Multicentric trials carry the disadvantage of including operations performed by many surgeons with different and very often limited experience, thus outweighing the advantage of the large number of patients included and weakening the strength of the conclusions drawn. Both meta-analyses were unable to find enough evidence for long-term outcomes on cancer recurrence and survival. Furthermore, data concerning lymph node retrieval that derive from comparative studies are lacking. A randomized trial comparing the outcomes after either laparoscopic or conventional open surgery in patients with rectal cancer was set up in three surgical units. In the present study, the adequacy of oncological clearance as depicted by the number of lymph nodes retrieved is discussed.

Methods

Patients

All patients with low rectal carcinoma were randomly allocated to undergo total mesorectal excision (TME) on an intention-to-cure basis by either the open (group A) or the laparoscopic (group B) approach, in three surgical units. Randomization was performed by computer-generated numbers. Collected data included patients' demographics, clinical and imaging characteristics of the tumor, neoadjuvant treatment if given, type of surgical resection and anastomosis if performed, and histopathologic reports on the extent of tumor invasion, status of lymph nodes retrieved (number, location in relation to the tumor and possible infiltration by the tumor) and final TNM staging.

Tumor Clinical Characteristics and Preoperative Staging

Only rectal tumors located within the distal 12 cm from the anal verge were included in the study. Digital examination and rigid sigmoidoscopy were applied to assess tumor extent at the periphery of the rectum, distance from the anal verge and fixation. An anterior component of the tumor was specifically mentioned, as this necessitated the administration of neoadjuvant treatment irrespective of the extent of invasion. Staging of the tumor was achieved by pelvic MRI in all cases and occasionally by endorectal ultrasound.

Patients with an anteriorly located T2–T4 tumor, a T3 tumor with a <5 mm free circumferential margin, lymph node involvement, venous invasion, and T4 or bulky locally advanced tumor were subjected to a high-dose radiotherapy and chemotherapy (total of 45 Gray and 5-fluorouracil per os over 5 weeks), followed by surgery 8–10 weeks later. Patients with tumors extending to the pelvic walls or organs were excluded from the study. Patients with anterior located T1, T2, and T3 tumors with a >5 mm free circumferential margin were given a preoperative short hypofractionated scheme of radiotherapy (total of 25 Gray over 5 days) followed by surgery 10–15 days later. The decision to perform either a low anterior resection of the rectum (LARR) with stapled colorectal anastomosis, or a LARR with intersphincteric resection and hand-sawn coloanal anastomosis, or an abdominoperineal resection (APR) was made prior to any downsizing of the tumor by the neoadjuvant treatment.

Surgical Techniques

All procedures were either performed or supervised by the most experienced surgeon. The first stage of the procedure, by either approach, involved ligation and division of the inferior mesenteric vein immediately below the Treitz ligament, and ligation and division of the inferior mesenteric artery at approximately 1 cm distal to its origin from the aorta, taking care to leave the hypogastric nerves intact behind, while clearing off the lymph nodes along the course of the vessel. Mobilization of the sigmoid and descending colon was carried out by the medial-to-lateral fashion of dissection, in between the two leaves of Toldt's fascia.

In case of the LARR, the 'holy plane' between the pelvic and rectal fasciae posterior to the rectum was entered and developed distally to the rectosacral ligament, which was sharply divided. The hypogastric nerves were safely left behind. The peritoneum at both sides of the upper part of the rectum was incised, and the two lines of incision met anteriorly on the crest of the peritoneal reflection, at 1–2 cm anteriorly to the cul-de-sac. The space anteriorly to the Denonvillier's fascia at the mid-rectum and posteriorly to the seminal vesicles and prostate in male or vagina in female was entered. The Denonvilliers' fascia was transversely incised as it becomes adherent to the prostatic apex in male, or at the level of distal transaction of the rectum in female. Laterally, the lateral ligaments of the rectum were divided on their medial part, in order to preserve the hypogastric nerves. In case of intersphincteric resection, the fascia covering the levator ani was incised and the space between the anal sphincters and the bowel wall was entered. If a part of rectal stump was left in situ above the levator ani musculature, it was completely denuded posterior from the tail of the distal mesorectum. The vertical transection of the rectum distal to the tumor was achieved with the use of a linear stapling device, and a stapled colorectal anastomosis was fashioned. When an intersphincteric resection of the rectum was performed, distal transaction was carried out transanally and the specimen was exteriorized through the anus, and a hand-sewn coloanal anastomosis followed. The distance of the anastomotic line from the anal verge was measured by on-table anoscopy. A covering ileostomy was fashioned in almost all cases.

In case of an APR, posterior dissection ended at the level of the rectosacral ligament. At the perineal stage, the excision was carried out widely on the skin and involved the ischirectal fat and most of the bulk of the lavatory ani, covered orally by a plate of fascia. The excised specimen should appear at its distal part in the form of a 'cylinder' rather than having a 'waist' between the tail of the mesorectum and the anal sphincters [26]. In most instances, the perineal gap was covered with a biological prosthetic material, and the perineal skin was sutured over it.

Histopathology Report on Lymph Nodes

All lymph nodes in the specimen should be identified, dissected and embedded. At first, the apical lymph nodes, adjacent to the point of ligation of the vascular pedicle are dissected. Thereafter, the mesentery is cut at the mesenteric edge of the bowel wall, avoiding removal of any area in which subserosal fat tissue may be involved by the carcinoma. The mesentery is divided into three levels: the level proximal to the tumor that involves mesenteric tissue at a radius of 1 cm, the intermediate level and the apical level. Then thin sections from each level are performed at 1-mm intervals, and examined by careful palpation. Any firm tissue remaining after gentle pressure is isolated and considered as lymph node and embedded separately. All the lymph nodes are embedded in totality, including those with large dimensions.

Four sections of each lymph node are examined after hematoxylin and eosin staining. Extramural tumor deposits measuring >3 mm are considered and counted as involved lymph nodes, even if no residual lymph node tissue can be identified.

Statistical Analysis

Statistical analysis was performed with the use of SPSS Version 11.5 software for Windows (SPSS, Chicago, Ill., USA). Values are expressed as median and range. Comparisons between the two groups of patients were made by applying either the Student t test or the Mann-Whitney U test for unpaired values, as appropriate. The χ^2 test was applied to compare differences in variables expressed in proportions. Differences were considered to be significant for p values <0.05.

Results

Thirty-nine patients (23 male) with a median age of 69 (41–85) years were allocated in group A and 34 (20 male) with a mean age of 72 (31–84) years in group B. Rectal tumors were located at a significantly higher level from the anal verge in group A than in group B (8 (1–12) cm vs. 6 (1–12) cm; p = 0.03). In 10 cases in group A and in 9 in group B, the rectal tumor involved the anterior rectal wall. Five cases in group A and 3 in group B had a T4 tumor. Ten patients in group A and 8 in group B had a T3 tumor in a distance <5 mm from the circumferential margin of the mesorectum (table 1). Fewer patients in group A had T3/T4 tumors than in group B group (61.54 vs. 72.72%), although the difference was not significant. Concerning the lymph nodes status, there were 24 N0, 10 N1, and 5 N2 cases in group A, and 28 N0, 3 N1 and 2 N2 cases in group B. Thus, based on preoperative staging, 17 patients in group A and 13 group B were given neoadjuvant treatment (group A: 4 short scheme radiation, 13 long scheme chemoradiation; group B: 3 short scheme radiation, 10 long scheme chemoradiation).

Table 1. Preoperative staging of the tumor (T) based on MRI of the pelvis

	Group A	Group B
T1	2	2
T2	13	7
T3	19 (10)	22 (8)
T4	5	3

The number of cases with a distance of <5 mm from the circumferential margin is shown in parentheses

Significantly more cases in group B had intersphincteric resection and abdominoperineal resection of the rectum than in group A (p = 0.04). Also, colorectal or anal anastomoses were significantly lower in group B than in group A (mean distance from dentate line: group B: 3.5 (1–4.5) cm vs. group A: 5.5 (1.5–8.5) cm; p < 0.001). Conceivably, a significantly larger number of patients after laparoscopy had a protecting ileostomy (p = 0.04) (table 2). There was one conversion of laparoscopy to open surgery (3%), because of tumor fixation to the right lateral pelvic wall. No specific technical difficulties nor greater blood loss were accounted in patients with neoadjuvant treatment after either approach, as compared to those without.

There was no significant difference in the total number of retrieved lymph nodes between groups (group A: 19.2 (5–45); group B: 19.2 (8–41) (p = 0.2)). Also, the numbers of regional, intermediate and apical lymph nodes did not differ significantly between groups. In 19 patients of group A and 23 of group B, lymph nodes had metastatic deposits (table 3).

Table 2. Operative details

	Group A	Group B
Total number of patients	39	34
Type of surgery		
Low anterior resection of rectum	34	22
Intersphincteric resection of rectum	1	5
Abdominoperineal resection of rectum	4	7
Distance of anastomosis from anal verge, cm (range)	5.5 (1.5–8.5)	4 (1–4.5)
Protective ileostomy, n (%)	10 (26)	14 (42)

Table 3. Histological characteristics of lymph nodes

	Group A	Group B
Lymph nodes, n (range)	19.2 (5–45)	19.2 (8–41)
Regional	3.9 (1–9)	3.7 (3–7)
Intermediate	13.9 (3–34)	14.4 (4–33)
Apical	1.5 (1–3)	1.3 (1–3)
Lymph node infiltration		
Positive	19	23
Negative	20	11

Discussion

Laparoscopy has been easily adopted for colon surgery, but is slowly gaining acceptance by the surgical community for rectal cancer. This is because of the initial concerns about adequacy of free resection margins and lymph node retrieval, while performing a TME for middle and low rectal cancer. Two recently published meta-analyses show that laparoscopic rectal cancer surgery may accomplish an oncological clearance of similar quality to the open approach [4, 5]. Of the 23 studies included in those meta-analyses, only 4 were randomized trials, 3 from a single institution with small number of patients [6–8] and 1 multicentric [9]. The evidence of adequate oncological clearance provided by those studies is rather weak, because of methodological drawbacks. In addition, an adequate oncological clearance for rectal cancer should be reflected in the long-term outcomes, namely local recurrence and survival. But again, existing evidence derived from the above studies is weak. This is because the large statistical power of multicenter trials is overwhelmed by the inhomogeneous adjuvant and neoadjuvant regimens applied by participating teams and the varying degree of experience of the surgeons practicing laparoscopic rectal surgery. Inadequate experience is illustrated at the conversion rate of laparoscopic resection of the rectum, which in the recently published multicenter CLASICC trial is as high as 34% [9]. On the contrary, the quality of surgery is high and the conversion rate very low in two published series of laparoscopic rectal resection, where only very experienced surgeons were involved [27, 28]. Also, recurrence and overall survival in these two series is similar to those reported by the best performers of the open approach [1, 2]. More homogenous comparative studies, namely prospective randomized trials conducted by a single experienced surgical team with a uniform updated oncological approach in terms of neoadjuvant and adjuvant treatment, will provide more solid evidence on the oncological safety of the laparoscopic approach for rectal cancer.

The meta-analysis by Aziz et al. [4] including 1,375 patients from 17 studies shows no significant differences in the proportion of patients with positive radial margins and the number of lymph nodes harvested between laparoscopic and open LARR or APR for rectal cancer surgery. Of the six studies reporting on lymph node retrieval included in the meta-analysis by Gao et al. [5], five report no difference in lymph node numbers removed with the specimen between the open and the laparoscopic resection of the rectum; in only one study by Araujo et al. [7], the number of lymph nodes retrieved by the open approach was significantly larger than that by laparoscopy.

Because it has been shown that many nodal metastases in colorectal cancer are found in small lymph nodes of <5 mm in diameter and that a minimum of 12–18 lymph nodes must be examined, a very careful search for lymph nodes must be performed [29, 30]. These criteria have been fulfilled at histology in the present study, the results of which showed no significant difference in the number of lymph nodes harvested by either the open or the laparoscopic approach. Furthermore, there were no differences whatsoever in the distribution of lymph nodes along the specimens; mean numbers of regional, intermediate and apical lymph nodes retrieved were similar between the two approaches. In this sense, laparoscopy seems to be of equal lymph node sampling capacity to the open approach, provided that all other aspects of an adequate quality of surgery are fulfilled by both approaches [31].

Rectal tumors in the laparoscopic group of the present study were located to a significantly lower level. This resulted in lower anastomoses and larger numbers of APR and intersphincteric resections undertaken compared to open surgery. However, cases with a threatened circumferential margin on preoperative imaging and final TN staging of the disease did not differ between the two approaches. None of these macroscopic or histological parameters seemed to affect the number of lymph nodes retrieved.

In conclusion, laparoscopic resection of the rectum achieves similar lymph node number retrieval with similar lymph node distribution along the resected specimen to the open approach, offering adequate sampling capacity. Lymph node clearance must be combined with other histological parameters so as to ensure that laparoscopic resection of the rectum is an approach that provides resection specimens of as high quality as the conventional open procedure.

References

1 Heald RJ, Husband EM, Ryall RDH: The mesorectum in rectal cancer surgery: the clue to pelvic recurrence? Br J Surg 1982;69:613–616.
2 Heald RJ, Karanjia ND: Results of radical surgery for rectal cancer. World J Surg 1992; 16: 848–857.
3 Dahlberg M, Glimelius B, Pahlman L: Changing strategy for rectal cancer is associated with improved outcome. Br J Surg 1999; 86:379–384.
4 Aziz O, Constantinides V, Tekkis PP, et al: Laparoscopic versus open surgery for rectal cancer: a meta-analysis. Ann Surg Oncol 2006;13:413–424.
5 Gao F, Cao YF, Chen LS: Meta-analysis of the short-term outcomes after laparoscopic resection for rectal cancer. Int J Colorectal Dis 2006;7:1–5.
6 Quah HM, Jayne DG, Eu KW, Seow-Choen F: Bladder and sexual dysfunction following laparoscopically assisted and conventional open mesorectal resection for rectal cancer. Br J Surg 2002;89:1551–1556.
7 Araujo SE, da Silva e Sousa AH Jr, de Campos FG, et al: Conventional approach versus laparoscopic abdominoperineal resection for rectal cancer treatment after neoadjuvant chemoradiation: results of a prospective randomized trial. Rev Hosp Clin Fac Med São Paolo 2003;58:133–140.
8 Breukink SO, Grond AJK, Pierie JPEN, Hoff C, Wiggers T, Meijerink WJHJ: Laparoscopic vs. open total mesorectal excision for rectal cancer. An evaluation of the mesorectum's macroscopic quality. Surg Endosc 2005;19:307–310.
9 Guillou PJ, Quirke P, Thorpe H, et al: Short-term endpoints of conventional versus laparoscopic assisted surgery in patients with colorectal cancer (MRC CLASICC trial): multicentre, randomised controlled trial. Lancet 2005;365:1718–1726.
10 Tate JJ, Kwok S, Dawson JW, et al: Prospective comparison of laparoscopic and conventional anterior resection. Br J Surg 1993;80: 1396–1398.
11 Darzi A, Lewis C, Menzies-Gow N, et al: Laparoscopic abdominoperineal excision of the rectum. Surg Endosc 1995;9:414–417.
12 Goh YC, Eu KW, Seow-Choen F: Early postoperative results of a prospective series of laparoscopic vs. open anterior resections for rectosigmoid cancers. Dis Colon Rectum 1997;40:776–780.
13 Leung KL, Kwok SP, Lau WY, et al: Laparoscopic-assisted resection of rectosigmoid carcinoma. Immediate and medium-term results. Arch Surg 1997;132:761–764.
14 Seow-Choen F, Eu KW, Ho YH, Leong AF: A preliminary comparison of a consecutive series of open versus laparoscopic abdominoperineal resection for rectal adenocarcinoma. Int J Colorectal Dis 1997;12:88–90.
15 Ramos JR, Petrosemolo RH, Valory EA, et al: Abdominoperineal resection: laparoscopic versus conventional. Surg Laparosc Endosc 1997;7:148–152.
16 Iroatulam AJ, Agachan F, Alabaz O, et al: Laparoscopic abdominoperineal resection for anorectal cancer. Am Surg 1998;64:12–18.
17 Fleshman JW, Wexner SD, Anvari M, et al: Laparoscopic vs. open abdominoperineal resection for cancer. Dis Colon Rectum 1999; 42:930–939.
18 Schwandner O, Schiedeck TH, Killaitis C, Bruch HP: A case-control-study comparing laparoscopic versus open surgery for rectosigmoidal and rectal cancer. Int J Colorectal Dis 1999;14:158–163.
19 Leung KL, Kwok SP, Lau WY, et al: Laparoscopic-assisted abdominoperineal resection for low rectal adenocarcinoma. Surg Endosc 2000;14:67–70.
20 Hartley JE, Mehigan BJ, Qureshi AE, et al: Total mesorectal excision: assessment of the laparoscopic approach. Dis Colon Rectum 2001;44: 315–321.
21 Baker RP, White EE, Titu L, et al: Does laparoscopic abdominoperineal resection of the rectum compromise long-term survival? Dis Colon Rectum 2002;45:1481–1485.
22 Anthuber M, Fuerst A, Elser F, et al: Outcome of laparoscopic surgery for rectal cancer in 101 patients. Dis Colon Rectum 2003; 46:1047–1053.

23 Feliciotti F, Guerrieri M, Paganini AM, et al: Long-term results of laparoscopic versus open resections for rectal cancer for 124 unselected patients. Surg Endosc 2003;17:1530–1535.
24 Vorob'ev GI, Shelygin IuA, Frolov SA, et al: Laparoscopic surgery of rectal cancer (comparative results of laparoscopic and open abdominal resection) (in Russian). Khirurgiia (Mosk) 2003;3:36–42.
25 Wu WX, Sun YM, Hua YB, Shen LZ: Laparoscopic versus conventional open resection of rectal carcinoma: a clinical comparative study. World J Gastroenterol 2004;10:1167–1170.
26 Radcliffe A: Can the results of anorectal (abdominoperineal resection) be improved: are circumferential resection margins too often positive? Colorectal Dis 2006;8:160–167.
27 Morino M, Parini U, Giraudo G, Salval M, Brachet Contul R, Garonne C: Laparoscopic total mesorectal excision: a consecutive series of 100 patients. Ann Surg 2003;237:335–342.
28 Leroy J, Jamali F, Forbes L, et al: Laparoscopic total mesorectal excision for rectal cancer surgery: long-term outcomes. Surg Endosc 2004;18:281–289.
29 Jass JR, Morson BC: Reporting colorectal cancer. J Clin Pathol 1987;40:1016–1023.
30 Carolyn C, Compton CA: The staging of colorectal Cancer: 2004 and beyond. Cancer J Clin 2004;54:295–308.
31 Nagtegaal ID, van de Velde CJ, van der Worp E, Kapiteijn E, Quirke P, van Krieken JH, Cooperative Clinical Investigators of the Dutch Colorectal Cancer Group: Macroscopic evaluation of rectal cancer resection specimen: clinical significance of the pathologist in quality control. J Clin Oncol 2002;20:1729–1734.

Original Article

Digestive Diseases

Dig Dis 2007;25:100–105
DOI: 10.1159/000099177

Irinotecan plus Weekly 5-Fluorouracil and Leucovorin as Salvage Treatment for Patients with Metastatic Colorectal Cancer: A Phase II Trial

J. Souglakos N. Vardakis N. Androulakis S. Kakolyris C. Kourousis
D. Mavroudis A. Pallis S. Agelaki K. Kalbakis V. Georgoulias

Department of Medical Oncology, University General Hospital of Heraklion, Greece

Key Words

Irinotecan · 5-Fluorouracil · Leucovorin · CPT-11/5-FU/LV (AIO schedule) · Metastatic colorectal cancer · Metastatic colorectal cancer, salvage treatment · Oxaliplatin

Abstract

Background: A phase II study was conducted to evaluate the toxicity and efficacy of irinotecan/5-fluorouracil/leucovorin (CPT-11/5-FU/LV (AIO schedule)) as salvage treatment in patients with metastatic colorectal cancer. ***Patients and Methods:*** 33 patients relapsing after oxaliplatin (L-OHP)-based first-line chemotherapy were enrolled. Their median age was 69 years, 20 (61%) patients were male, and performance status (WHO) was 0, 1, and 2 in 15, 16 and 2 patients respectively; prior surgery 20 (61%) patients; adjuvant chemotherapy 11 (33%) patients, and adjuvant radiotherapy 6 (18%) patients. The number of metastatic sites was 1, 2, and ≥3 in 11, 11, and 11 patients, respectively. CPT-11 was administered on day 1 at the dose of 80 mg/m^2 in 30–90 min infusion and LV (500 mg/m^2) on the same day as a 2-hour infusion followed by 5-FU (2,600 mg/m^2/day) as a 22-hour infusion on day 1 for 6 subsequent weeks. The regimen was repeated every 7 weeks. ***Results:*** All patients were evaluable for toxicity and for response. Complete response was achieved in 2 patients (6%) and partial response in 4 patients (12%) (RR 18%, CI 5.95–35.43%); 13 patients (40%) had stable disease, and 14 (42%) progressive disease. After a median follow-up period of 9 months, the median duration of response was 5 months, the median time to progression 7.5 months, and OS 14 months. Grade 3–4 neutropenia occurred in 13 patients (39%), febrile neutropenia in 3 (9%), grade 2 anemia in 11 (33%), grade 4 thrombocytopenia in 1 (3%). Grade 3–4 diarrhea occurred in 12 patients (36%), grade 3–4 neurotoxicity in 3 (9%), and grade 3 asthenia in 4 (12%). No treatment-related deaths occurred. The median dose intensity was 85% for CPT-11, and 88% for 5-FU and LV. ***Conclusions:*** The combination of weekly CPT-11 and infusional 5-FU/LV is an active and relatively well-tolerated regimen as salvage treatment in MCC.

Introduction

Colorectal cancer is one of the most common cancers in developed countries, after breast cancer in females and lung and prostate cancer in males. In Europe, the predicted annual incidence is approximately 150,000 new cases, with mortality of about 80,000–95,000 [1]. Similarly, in the USA, colon cancer alone causes 56,000 deaths and 130,000 new cases every year [2].

KARGER

Fax +41 61 306 12 34
E-Mail karger@karger.ch
www.karger.com

0257–2753/07/0251–0100$23.50/0

Accessible online at:
www.karger.com/ddi

Dr. Vassilis Georgoulias, MD, PhD
Department of Medical Oncology, University General Hospital
PO Box 1352
GR–71110 Heraklion (Greece)
Tel. +30 81 392 747, Fax +30 81 392 802, E-Mail georsec@med.uch.gr

Despite macroscopically curative surgical resection in 70–80% of cases, half of those colorectal cancer patients will develop recurrence (mostly metastatic recurrence) and will die of the disease [2]. For more than 40 years, 5-fluorouracil (5-FU) was the only cytotoxic agent sharing a significant activity in advanced colorectal cancer. Until recently, the standard therapy for metastatic colorectal cancer (MCC) was 5-FU, modulated by calcium folinate (leucovorin (LV)), which typically achieves a median survival of 10–14 months [3, 4]. Oxaliplatin (L-OHP), a new diaminocyclohexane-platinum analog, has also shown significant activity in advanced colorectal cancer [5]. Two randomized trials have compared the combination of L-OHP with 5-FU/LV given either chronomodulated or in accordance with the de Gramont schedule, with that of the same 5-FU/LV regimen alone as first-line treatment of MCC [6, 7]. The addition of L-OHP to 5-FU/LV significantly improved the overall response rate and median time to tumor progression, but not the median survival time.

Many patients with advanced colorectal cancer are candidates for additional chemotherapy after failure of fluoropyrimidine-based chemotherapy. The topoisomerase I inhibitor irinotecan (CPT-11) has been proven to be of particular value in this treatment setting. Significant survival advantage and a clinical benefit were observed when CPT-11 compared to best supportive care alone [8] or continuous 5-FU infusion [9]. CPT-11 is now considered standard second-line treatment in this patient population.

In the last few years, evidence has accumulated that a prolonged infusion of 5-FU may improve the tumor response rate and time to tumor progression when compared with 5-FU bolus regimen [10]. Additionally, the German Association of Medical Oncology (AIO), in a phase I multicenter trial in MCC, demonstrated an overall response rate of 64% using a weekly time-six schedule of CPT-11 (80 mg/m^2) and high-dose LV (500 mg/m^2) followed by infusional 5-FU (2,600 mg/m^2) [11].

Schedule-dependent cytotoxic interactions for the combination of thymidylate synthetase inhibitors with SN-38 have been reported in in vitro models [12]. This data on human colon tumor cell lines suggested a synergistic antitumor effect for the two drugs if CPT-11 preceded 5-FU. Moreover, these data suggest that CPT-11, and 5-FU are active drugs in the treatment of MCC, sharing different mechanisms of action and non-overlapping toxicities.

Based on these data, a phase II study was conducted in order to assess the efficacy and safety of CPT-11 in combination with LV-modulated infusional 5-FU administered according to the AIO schedule in patients with advanced colorectal cancer refractory or resistant to (CI) 5-FU/LV and L-OHP.

Patients and Methods

Eligibility Criteria

From April 1999 to March 2001, 33 patients with histologically proven metastatic adenocarcinoma of the colon or rectum were enrolled. All patients had received L-OHP-based chemotherapy for metastatic disease. Patients who had presented tumor progression under treatment or within 3 months from the end of chemotherapy were considered as refractory to L-OHP-based first-line chemotherapy. Patients with operable metastatic disease were excluded from the study. Other eligibility criteria were: age 18–75 years, performance status (according WHO) 0–2; at least one bidimensionally measurable lesion of ≥2 cm; a life expectancy of at least 3 months; adequate hematologic parameters (absolute neutrophil count ≥1.5 × 10^9/l and platelets ≥100 × 10^9/l); creatinine 1.25 or less times the upper limit of normal; total bilirubin 1.25 or less times the upper limit of normal; aspartate aminotransferase and alanine aminotransferase 3.0 or less times the upper limit of normal; absence of active infection of malnutrition; absence of a second primary tumor. Patients treated with palliative radiotherapy had to have measurable metastatic disease outside the irradiation fields. Patients with severe cardiac dysfunction, liver metastases involving more than 50% of the liver parenchyma, or with chronic diarrheic syndrome, or prior irradiation affecting more than 30% of the bone marrow were not eligible. The study was approved by the ethics and scientific committees of all institutes. All patients gave written informed consent in order to participate in the study.

Chemotherapy

CPT-11 was given at a dose of 80 mg/m^2 as 30–90-min intravenous infusion on day 1. LV was given at a dose of 500 mg/m^2 as a 2-hour intravenous infusion, followed by 5-FU at the dose of 2,600 mg/m^2 as a 22-hour continuous infusion on day 1. Routine antiemetic prophylaxis with a 5-hydroxytryptamine-3 receptor antagonist was used. Treatment was administered every week for 6 consecutive weeks in cycles of 7 weeks (1 week rest). Treatment was continued until disease progression, the appearance of unacceptable toxicity, or patient's consent withdrawal.

Patients were assessed for toxicity before each 2-week cycle using the common toxicity criteria of the National Cancer Institute. Chemotherapy was delayed until recovery if neutrophils decreased to <1.5 × 10^9/l or platelets decreased to <100 × 10^9/l or for significant persisting non-hematologic toxicity. CPT-11 was administered according to the guidelines used for CPT-11 monotherapy, including recommendations for the use of atropine and loperamide. Doses of all drugs were reduced by 15% in subsequent cycles in case of grade 3–4 neutropenia, grade 3–4 thrombocytopenia lasting for more than 3 days or in case of febrile neutropenia. No prophylactic administration of granulocyte colony-stimulating factor was allowed. Doses of CPT-11 and 5-FU were reduced by 15% in subsequent cycles in case of grade 3–4 diarrhea. The 5-FU dose was reduced after grade 3–4 stomatitis or if dermatitis occurred.

Evaluation

Pretreatment evaluation included a detailed medical history and physical examination, a complete blood cell count with differential and platelet counts, whole blood chemistry, determination of serum levels of carcinoembryonic antigen and computed tomography (CT) scans of the chest and abdomen. Pretreatment evaluation had to be performed within 2 weeks prior to study entry. In addition, patients were clinically assessed and routine biochemical tests were performed before each treatment cycle. Response to treatment was assessed after two 7-week cycles or sooner if clinically indicated with the same method using a baseline evaluation.

WHO criteria were used to assess tumor response. Complete response was defined as the complete disappearance of all clinically assessable diseases for at least 4 weeks, and partial response was defined as a decrease of at least 50% of the sum of the products of the diameters of measurable lesions for at least 4 weeks. CT scans were performed at least 4 weeks later to confirm a response. Stable disease was defined as a decrease of less than 50% or an increase of less than 25% of measurable lesions, and progressive disease was defined as an increase of at least 25% of measurable lesion or the appearance of new malignant lesion(s).

The duration of response was measured from the first documentation of response to disease progression. The time to tumor progression was determined by the interval between the initiation of treatment and the date when disease progression was first documented. The follow-up time was measured from the day of first treatment administration to the last contact or death.

Statistical Consideration

This was a two-step phase II study; if an objective response rate more than 15% was observed in the first 15 patients, an additional 15 patients should be enrolled. The probability of survival was estimated by the Kaplan-Meier method [13], and the confidence intervals for response rates were calculated using methods for exact binomial confidence intervals [14]. The Global Health Status/Quality of Life (QOL) mean scale score at the start and end of chemotherapy was the major endpoint for the QOL assessment.

Results

Patients Characteristics

Between June 1999 and April 2001, 33 pretreated patients with metastatic colorectal were enrolled in the study. Their median age was 69 years, and 20 of them (61%) were males; 31 (94%) of the patients had PS 0–1, and the median number of involved sites was 2 per patient. Eleven patients (33%) had progressed and 12 (36%) failed to respond to L-OHP + 5-FU/LV chemotherapy regimen, while 10 (31%) had initially responded but progressed within 3 months after the completion of their treatment. The median interval between previous treatment and initiation of this regimen was 5.5 (range 1–9) months. The patients' characteristics are shown in table 1. All patients were evaluable for toxicity and for response to treatment.

Table 1. Patients' characteristics

	Patients	%
Number of patients enrolled	33	
Age		
Median	69	
Range	47–75	
Sex		
Male	20	61
Female	13	39
Performance status (WHO)		
0	15	45
1	16	49
2	2	6
Primary tumor		
Colon	9	27
Sigmoid	13	39
Rectum	11	34
Sites of disease		
Local abdominal mass	10	30
Liver	25	76
Lung	12	55
Lymph nodes	9	27
Bone	2	6
Other	8	24
Number of metastatic sites		
1	11	33
2	11	33
≥3	11	33

Efficacy

Complete response was observed in 2 (6%) patients and partial response in 4 (13%) patients resulting in an overall response rate of 19% (95% CI: 5.45–33.26%) (intention-to-treat analysis); moreover, 13 (42%) patients had stable disease and 12 (39%) progressive disease. One of the patients who responded was refractory to FOLFOX4, while the other 4 were resistant. The response rate was 57% in lymph nodes, 65% in liver metastases, 75% in lung metastases, and 40% in local disease. The median duration of response was 5 (range 2.5–17.5) months, while the median time to tumor progression was 7.5 (range 4.5–19.5) months. After a median follow-up period of 18 (range 8.5–29.5) months, the overall median survival time was 14 (range 2–19.5) months; the probability for 1-year survival was 56.31% (fig. 1), and 18 patients are still alive at the time of the present analysis.

Toxicity

Diarrhea and neutropenia were the most common toxic effects of the combination. The hematologic and

Table 2. Toxicity of the CPT-11/5-FU/LV combination in all patients and all cycles

	Grade 1		Grade 2		Grade 3		Grade 4	
	n	%	n	%	n	%	n	%
Hematologic toxicity								
Neutropenia	3	9	7	21	11	33	2	6
Anemia	19	58	11	33	1	3	–	–
Thrombocytopenia	11	33	1	3	–	–	1	3
Febrile neutropenia	–	–	1	3	–	–	2	6
Non-hematologic toxicity								
Nausea	5	15	6	18	–	–	–	–
Diarrhea	7	21	6	18	9	27	3	9
Mucositis	6	18	–	–	–	–	1	3
Neurotoxicity	7	21	3	9	4	12	1	3
Fatigue	10	30	7	21	4	12	–	–
Cutaneous	3	10	–	–	–	–	–	–
Infections without concomitant grade 3–4 neutropenia	–	–	2	6	1	3	–	–

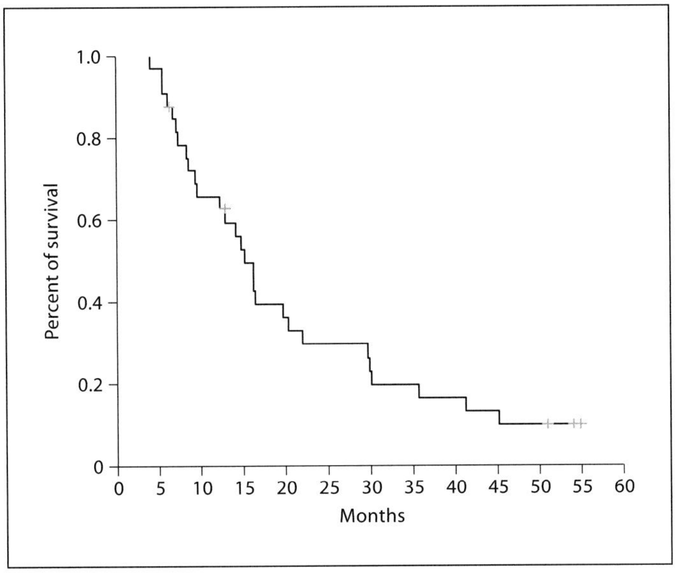

Fig. 1. Kaplan-Meier survival curve for the 33 patients receiving the CPT-11/5-FU/LV combination.

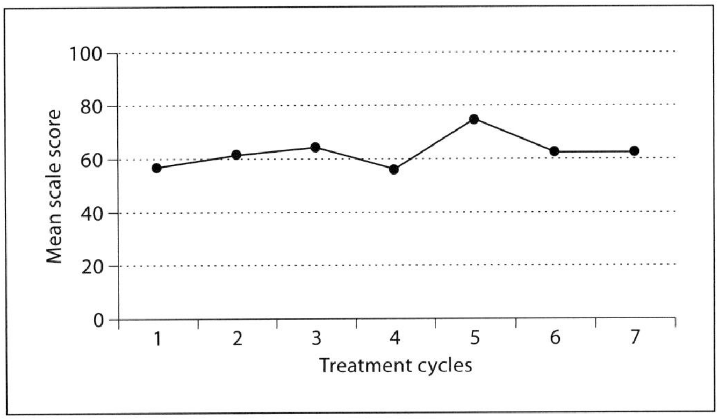

Fig. 2. Variation of the Global Health Status mean scale score during treatment with the triplet combination.

non-hematologic toxicity of the regimen is presented in table 2. Neutropenia grade 3 or 4 was observed in 13 (39%) patients, while 3 (9%) patients developed febrile neutropenia requiring hospitalization and treatment with intravenous antibiotics. Grade 3 anemia occurred in 1 (3%) patient. Thrombocytopenia grade 3–4 was observed in 1 (3%) patient. Grade 3 or 4 diarrhea developed in 12 (36%) patients and grade 3 fatigue in 4 (12%). Mucositis grade 4 was observed in 1 (3%) patient. Neurosensory toxicity was observed in 15 (45%) patients and reached grade 3 in 4 (12%) patients and grade 4 in 1 (3%) patient. Three (9%) patients developed infection without concomitant grade 3 or 4 neutropenia, but only 1 (3%) was hospitalized and treated with intravenous antibiotics. The other grade 3 or 4 toxicities were infrequent. None of the patients developed hand-foot syndrome. Four treatment-related admissions to the hospital were reported, 3 for diarrhea grade 3 or 4 and 1 for diarrhea and grade 4 neutropenia. There were no treatment-related deaths.

Table 3. Relief of symptoms

	Improvement	Stable	Worsening
Pain (n = 22)	14	3	5
Bleeding (n = 3)	3	–	–
Fever (n = 4)	4	–	–

Compliance to Treatment

129 courses of chemotherapy were administered (median 3 courses per patient; range 2–8). 20 (16%) courses were delayed for a median of 5 (range 1–9) days. Hematologic toxicity was the reason for treatment delay in 7 (35%) courses, non-hematologic toxicity in 3 (15%) courses, while 10 (50%) courses were delayed due to reasons unrelated to treatment or disease. The median interval between cycles was 51 (range 49–57) days. Dose reduction was required in 19 (15%) cycles because of hematologic (7 cycles; 37%) and non-hematologic toxicity (12 cycles; 63%). G-CSF was administered in 13 (7.3) cycles for the treatment of severe neutropenia. The relative dose intensity was 85% for CPT-11, and 88% for 5-FU and LV.

Quality of Life and Relief of Symptoms

184 questionnaires were completed from 33 patients. The rate of form return was 82%. The Global Health Status/QOL mean scale score remained unchanged, with a slight improvement during the treatment (fig. 2). 29 (88%) patients had at least one disease-related symptom at baseline. 22 patients had presented with abdominal pain (table 3). Pain relief (decrease of the drug doses or discontinuation of analgesic therapy) was observed in 14 (64%) patients. One of the patients had achieved a complete remission, while 3 had presented with partial response and 10 had present stable disease. In 3 patients with gastrointestinal bleeding and 4 with fever, complete resolution of their symptoms was observed.

Discussion

Salvage treatment for pretreated patients with advanced colorectal cancer is a particularly difficult task, depending on the type and duration of front-line treatment. Many patients with oligosymptomatic disease and good performance status require palliative treatment for the control of disease-related symptoms and, probably, the prolongation of survival. However, the development of L-OHP and CPT-11 created additional treatment options for patients with refractory or resistant to 5-FU/LV colorectal cancer [8–9, 15–17].

In the present study, the combination of CPT-11 + 5-FU/LV (AIO schedule) resulted in 19% objective responses and 61% tumor growth control in a group of patients with advanced colorectal cancer resistant or refractory to L-OHP + 5-FU/LV. However, it is still unclear whether the observed efficacy of the CPT-11 + 5-FU/LV is due to CPT-11 alone or to the combination of CPT-11 + 5-FU/LV. Furthermore, patients treated with CPT-11 + 5-FU/LV salvage chemotherapy presented a median time to tumor progression of 7.5 months and an overall median survival of 14 months after the initiation of the CPT-11 + 5-FU/LV regimen which are higher than those observed with CPT-11 monotherapy given as second line [8, 9, 18]. However, it is still unclear whether this salvage regimen may confer a survival benefit in patients with refractory or resistant advanced colorectal cancer to L-OHP-based chemotherapy and a prospective randomized study is requited to answer this question.

Recently, a multicenter randomized trial was performed in France [18]. The patients were treated with FOLFIRI as first-line chemotherapy followed by FOLFOX after disease progression, or with the opposite schedule (FOLFOX followed by FOLFIRI). The results showed similar response rates and median survival. Although progression was 3 months longer when the FOLFIRI regimen was used for the first time, fewer patients discontinued the treatment and more patients received second-line chemotherapy. In addition, the response rate was proven to be better when FOLFOX was administered as second-line treatment in comparison to FOLFIRI.

The toxicity profile of the combination of CPT-11 with LV/FU was relatively mild. As expected, the main toxicities were neutropenia and diarrhea. Grade 3–4 neutropenia was observed in 13 (39%) patients; however, febrile neutropenia occurred only in 3 (9%) patients. G-CSF was used in 13 (7.3%) cycles for the treatment of febrile of severe persistent neutropenia. Thrombocytopenia grade 4 was observed in 1 (3%) patient. No patient required red blood cell or platelet transfusions. Grade 3–4 diarrhea occurred in 12 (36%) patients and grade 3 fatigue in 4 (12%). Mucositis grade 4 was observed in 1 (3%) patient. Neurosensory toxicity was observed in 15 (45%) patients and reached grade 3 in 4 (12%) patients and grade 4 in 1 (3%) patient. This high incidence of neurotoxicity was a consequence of prior therapy with L-OHP. The toxicity profile of the combination was similar to that observed in previous studies [11].

In summary, the results of the present study demonstrate that the combination of weekly CPT-11 with high-dose LV and 5-FU in a 24-hour continuous infusion (AIO schedule) is a relatively active and well-tolerated salvage treatment for patients with refractory or resistant to L-OHP + 5-FU/LV MCC, although a randomized trial provided results that show favorable efficacy and toxicity profile when the combination of CPT-11 and 5-FU/LV is administered as first-line treatment and the L-OHP/5-FU/LV combination as salvage chemotherapy. A large randomized trial is needed to establish the possible benefit of CPT-11 combinations as salvage treatment in patients with advanced colorectal cancer.

Acknowledgements

This study was partially supported by the Cretan Association for Biomedical Research (CABR). Drs J. Souglakos and N. Vardakis are recipients of a CABR clinical fellowship.

References

1 Black RJ, Bray F, Ferlay J, et al: Cancer incidence and mortality in the European Union: cancer registry data and estimates of national incidence for 1990. Eur J Cancer 1997;33:1075–107.
2 American Cancer Society: Cancer facts and figures – 2000. Atlanta, ACS, 2000.
3 The Advanced Colorectal Cancer Meta-Analysis Project: Modulation of fluorouracil by leucovorin in patients with advanced colorectal cancer: evidence in terms of response rate. J Clin Oncol 1992;10:896–903.
4 Kohne CH, Schoffski P, Wilke H, et al: Effective biomodulation by leucovorin of high-dose infusion fluorouracil given as a weekly 24-hour infusion: results of a randomized trial in patients with advanced colorectal cancer. J Clin Oncol 1998;16:418–26.
5 Bleiberg H: Oxaliplatin: a new reality in colorectal cancer. Br J Cancer 1998;77(suppl 4):1S–3S.
6 Giacchetti S, Perpoint B, Zidani R, et al: Phase III multicenter randomized trial of oxaliplatin added to chronomodulated fluorouracil-leucovorin as first-line treatment of metastatic colorectal cancer J Clin Oncol 2000;18:136–147.
7 De Gramont A, Figer A, Seymour M, et al: Leucovorin and fluorouracil with or without oxaliplatin as first-line treatment in advanced colorectal cancer. J Clin Oncol 2000; 18:2938–2947.
8 Cunningham D, Pyrhonen S, James R, et al: Randomized trial of irinotecan plus supportive care versus supportive care alone after fluorouracil failure for patients with metastatic colorectal cancer. Lancet 1998;352: 1413–1418.
9 Rougier P, van Cutsem E, Bajetta E, et al: Randomised trial of irinotecan versus fluorouracil by continuous infusion after fluorouracil failure in patients with metastatic colorectal cancer. Lancet 1998;352:1407–1412.
10 De Gramont A, Bosset JF, Milan C, et al: Randomized trial comparing monthly low-dose leucovorin and fluorouracil bolus with bimonthly high-dose leucovorin and fluorouracil bolus plus continuous infusion for advanced colorectal cancer: A French intergroup study. J Clin Oncol 1997;14:808–815.
11 Vanhoefer U, Harstrick A, Kohne CH, et al: Phase I study of a weekly schedule of irinotecan, high-dose leucovorin and infusional fluorouracil as first-line chemotherapy in patients with advanced colorectal cancer. J Clin Oncol 1999;17:907–913.
12 Fischel JL, Rostagno P, Etienne MC, et al: Optimal combination between irinotecan, oxaliplatin and fluorouracil-folinic acid: experimental data on human colorectal cell lines. Proc Am Assoc Cancer Res 1999;40: 589, abstr 3882.
13 Kaplan EL, Meier P: Non-parametric estimation from incomplete observations. J Am Stat Assoc 1959;53:457–481.
14 Cox DR: The Analysis of Binary Data. London, Methnen, 1970.
15 Machover D, Diaz-Rubio E, de Gramont A, et al: Two consecutive phase II studies of oxaliplatin for treatment of patients with advanced colorectal carcinoma who were resistant to previous treatment with fluoropyrimidines. Ann Oncol 1996;6:95–98.
16 Saltz LB, Douillard J, Pirotta N, et al: Combined analysis of two phase III randomized trials comparing irinotecan, flourouracil, leucovorin vs. flourouracil alone as first-line treatment of metastatic colorectal cancer. Proc Am Soc Clin Oncol 2000;19:242, abstr 938.
17 Douillard JY, Cunningham D, Roth AD, et al: Irinotecan combined with fluorouracil compared with fluorouracil alone as first-line treatment for metastatic colorectal cancer: a multicenter randomized trial. Lancet 2000;355:1041–1047.
18 Ulrich-Pur H, Kornek GV, Fiebiger W, et al: Multicenter phase II trial of dose fractionated irinotecan with advanced colorectal cancer failed oxaliplatin-based first-line combination chemotherapy. Ann Oncol 2001;12:1269–1272.
19 Tournigand C, Louvet C, Quinaux E, et al: FOLFIRI followed by FOLFOX vs. FOLFOX followed by FOLFIRI in metastatic colorectal cancer: final results of a phase III study. Proc Am Soc Clin Oncol 2001;20:124, abstr 494.

Digestive Diseases

Author Index Vol. 25, No. 1, 2007

Subject Index Vol. 25, No. 1, 2007

KARGER

Fax +41 61 306 12 34
E-Mail karger@karger.ch
www.karger.com

Accessible online at:
www.karger.com/ddi